O P L
OXFORD PSYCHIATRY LIBRARY

Addiction

O P L
OXFORD PSYCHIATRY LIBRARY

Addiction

SECOND EDITION

David J. Nutt
The Edmond J. Safra Chair in Neuropsychopharmacology,
Centre for Neuropsychopharmacology,
Division of Brain Sciences, Department of Medicine,
Imperial College London, United Kingdom

Liam J. Nestor
Centre for Neuropsychopharmacology,
Division of Brain Sciences, Department of Medicine,
Imperial College London, United Kingdom

OXFORD
UNIVERSITY PRESS

OXFORD
UNIVERSITY PRESS

Great Clarendon Street, Oxford, OX2 6DP,
United Kingdom

Oxford University Press is a department of the University of Oxford.
It furthers the University's objective of excellence in research, scholarship,
and education by publishing worldwide. Oxford is a registered trade mark of
Oxford University Press in the UK and in certain other countries

The moral rights of the authors have been asserted
First Edition published in 2013
Second Edition published in 2018

Impression: 1

Published in the United States of America by Oxford University Press
198 Madison Avenue, New York, NY 10016, United States of America

British Library Cataloguing in Publication Data

Data available

Library of Congress Control Number: 2018937424

ISBN 978-0-19-879774-6

Printed in Great Britain by
Ashford Colour Press Ltd, Gosport, Hampshire

Preface

Substance addiction is conceived to involve a loss of self-control. Despite their best efforts and expressed preferences to remain abstinent, substance addiction populations often appear incapable of exerting sufficient control over their substance urges, their substance-seeking and substance-taking behaviours. The origins of substance addiction appear to be related to the long-term pharmacological effects of substances on an already, potentially genetically compromised set of neural circuits in the brain. There are credible theories regarding the initiation of substance abuse (e.g. a reward deficiency syndrome, impulsivity/impaired cognitive control, stress) whose antecedents are most likely to involve interactions between several neurotransmitter systems (e.g. dopamine, endorphins, GABA, glutamate) in the brain. This appears to be supported, to some degree, by the potential efficacy of some pharmacotherapies (e.g. agonists/antagonists at dopamine, endorphin, GABA, and glutamate receptors) that have been shown to increase the likelihood of substance abstinence and prevent relapse. Further research is required, however, in an attempt fully to define the neurochemistry of important behavioural components of substance addiction (e.g. craving, impulsivity) that feature prominently in substance use disorders, particularly with respect to substance relapse after significant periods of protracted abstinence.

The following volume will attempt to inform clinicians and other healthcare professionals about some of the more fundamental psychological, neurobiological, and pharmacological concepts that are applicable to the treatment of substance abuse and addiction. The following volume will place particular emphasis on reporting and discussing the seminal findings of human neuroscience research in substance addiction and clinical trials in different substance addiction populations.

David J. Nutt
Liam J. Nestor

Contents

Symbols and abbreviations

~	approximately
β	beta
%	percent
$\leq$	equal to or less than
3-HC	3'-hydroxycotinine
5-HT	5-hydroxytryptomine
A118G	arginine (A) to glycine (G) substitution at position 118 of exon 1
A&E	Accident and Emergency
ACG	anterior cingulate gyrus
ACh	acetylcholine
ADHD	attention deficit hyperactive disorder
AMPA	α-amino-3-hydroxy-5-methyl-4-isoxazolepropionic acid
Amyg	amygdala
ARS	Alcohol Rating Scale
ATP	adenosine triphosphate
AUD	alcohol-use disorder
BED	binge-eating disorder
BPND	parametric binding potential
BrAC	breath alcohol concentration
C-11	carbon 11
Ca^{2+}	calcium
cAMP	cyclic adenosine monophosphate
CB1	cannabinoid 1 receptor
CEQ	Cocaine Effects Questionnaire
CI	confidence interval
Cl^-	chloride
CIWA-Ar	Clinical Institute Withdrawal Assessment for Alcohol-revised
DA	dopamine
DALY	disability-adjusted life-year
DAT	dopamine transporter
DCS	D-cycloserine
DIAZ	diazepam
DLPFC	dorsolateral prefrontal cortex
dOR	delta opioid receptor
D1R	dopamine 1 receptor

D2R	dopamine 2 receptor
DS	dorsal striatum
DSM	*Diagnostic and Statistical Manual of Mental Disorders*
DXM	dextromethorphan
fMRI	functional magnetic resonance imaging
g	gram
GABA	gamma-aminobutyric acid
GABA-T	GABA-transaminase
GAD	glutamate decarboxylase
GHB	gammahydroxybutyrate
GHS-R	growth hormone secretagogue receptor
GLP-1	glucagon-like peptide-1
HIP	hippocampus
HR	hazard ratio
ICD	International Classification of Diseases and Health Problems
iv	intravenous
K^+	potassium
K	ketamine
kg	kilogram
kOR	kappa opioid receptor
LDTg	lateral dorsal tegmental nucleus
LSD	lysergic acid diethylamide
LTD	long-term depression
LTP	long-term potentiation
MA	methamphetamine
MDMA	3,4-methylenedioxy-*N*-methamphetamine
MFG	middle frontal gyrus
mg	milligram
Mg^{2+}	magnesium
mGluR	metabotropic glutamate receptor
min	minute
mm	millimetre
MOA	monoamine oxidase
mOR	mu opioid receptor
MP	methylphenidate
MRI	magnetic resonance imaging
Na^+	sodium
NAC	N-acetylcysteine

NAcc	nucleus accumbens
nAChRs	nicotinic acetylcholine receptors
NBM	nucleus basalis of Meynert
NMDA	N-methyl-D-aspartate
N_2O	nitric oxide
OFC	orbitofrontal cortex
OPRM1	opioid receptor mu 1
p	probability
PACS	Penn Alcohol Craving Scale
PCP	phencyclidine
PET	positron emission tomography
PFC	prefrontal cortex
PO	per os (by way of mouth)
PTSD	post-traumatic stress disorder
RDS	reward deficiency syndrome
ROI	region of interest
SADD	Short Alcohol Dependence Data
SEM	standard error of the mean
SN	substantia nigra
SR	slow release
SSRI	selective serotonin reuptake inhibitor
VAS	visual analogue scale
VLPFC	ventrolateral prefrontal cortex
VP	ventral pallidum
VS	ventral striatum
VTA	ventral tegmental area
WHO	World Health Organization
xc−	cystine-glutamate exchange
Zn^{2+}	zinc

What is addiction?

- Addiction is a brain disease.
- Addiction is a chronic relapsing disorder.
- Addiction involves the chronic pharmacological actions of substances in the brain.
- There are different types of addiction (e.g. alcohol, cocaine).
- Individuals may be more vulnerable to addiction than others.
- Endophenotypes of addiction may facilitate diagnosis and treatment.
- Addiction may involve numerous factors (e.g. social, biological).
- Addiction does not happen immediately.
- There are stages of addiction (e.g. preoccupation, loss of control).
- There are also 'non-substance' behavioural addictions (e.g. gambling).
- Limited use of addictive drugs is clinically distinct from addiction.

1.1 Introduction

From the Latin word *addictio* (enslaved), 'addiction' is a concept that has been subject to much debate for some considerable time. At its origin, 'addiction' simply referred to 'giving over', being 'highly devoted', or engaging in behaviour habitually, with positive or negative implications. Subsequent and more modern views of addiction to substances were framed around observations that those afflicted experienced strong, overpowering urges, which were conceived to be more disease-like in their origins.

Substance addiction is now defined as a chronic relapsing disorder characterized by: (1) compulsion to seek and take the substance, (2) loss of control in limiting substance intake, and (3) the emergence of a negative emotional state (e.g. dysphoria, anxiety, irritability) reflecting a motivational withdrawal syndrome when access to the substance is prevented (defined as substance dependence by the *Diagnostic and Statistical Manual of Mental Disorders* (DSM) of the American Psychiatric Association). According to DSM, there are seven main criteria for substance dependence (see Box 1.1).

Importantly, the occasional, but limited use of addictive substances is clinically distinct from escalated substance use, loss of control over substance intake, and the emergence of chronic compulsive substance-seeking that characterizes addiction.

> **Box 1.1** The criteria for substance dependence according to DSM
>
> (1) Tolerance, as defined by either of the following:
>   (a) A need for markedly increased amounts of the substance to achieve intoxication or desired effect.
>   (b) Markedly diminished effect with continued use of the same amount of the substance.
> (2) Withdrawal, as manifested by either of the following:
>   (a) The characteristic withdrawal syndrome for the substance (refer to Criteria A or B of the criteria sets for withdrawal from specific substances).
>   (b) The same (or a closely related) substance is taken to relieve or avoid withdrawal symptoms.
> (3) The substance is often taken in larger amounts or over a longer period than was intended.
> (4) There is a persistent desire to use the substance or unsuccessful efforts to cut down or control substance use.
> (5) A great deal of time is spent in activities necessary to obtain the substance (such as visiting multiple doctors or driving long distances), use the substance (such as chain smoking), or recover from its effects.
> (6) Important social, occupational, or recreational activities are given up or reduced because of substance use.
> (7) The substance use is continued despite knowledge of having a persistent or recurrent physical or psychological problem that is likely to have been caused or exacerbated by the substance.
>
> Source data from *Diagnostic and Statistical Manual of Mental Disorders (DSM-5)*, 2013, American Psychiatric Association

From modern-day psychological and pharmacological perspectives, substance addiction (including alcohol) may be seen as a manifestation of the long-term pharmacological actions of these substances on the receptor mechanisms of the brain. Evidence, however, is beginning to emerge that non-substance (i.e. behavioural) addictions, such as pathological gambling, show strong behavioural and neural similarities to substance addiction (see Box 1.2).

It is also surmised that some individuals may be more susceptible to substance addiction. This susceptibility may be due to abnormal receptor mechanisms in the brain which have been genetically inherited (i.e. a neurobiological predisposition). Substances of addiction exacerbate this predisposition. The development and emergence of substance addiction, however, may involve many factors— biological (i.e. genetics), social (e.g. socio-economic background), method of

Box 1.2 Substance and behavioural addictions

Substance addictions

- Alcohol
- Tobacco
- Opioids (like heroin)
- Prescription drugs (sedatives, hypnotics, or anxiolytics—like sleeping pills and tranquillizers)
- Cocaine
- Cannabis (marijuana)
- Amphetamines (like methamphetamine, known as crystal meth)
- Hallucinogens
- Inhalants
- Phencyclidine (known as PCP or angel dust)

Behavioural addictions

- Gambling
- Shopping
- Sex
- Internet

administration (e.g. intravenous, oral). Furthermore, these factors are unlikely to be independent, instead interacting with one another at different points in the addiction trajectory.

The emergence of endophenotypes may also be of relevance to the development and treatment of addiction disorders. The endophenotype may be neurophysiological, cognitive, or neuropsychological. Endophenotypes are present before addiction onset and in individuals with heritable risk for addiction (e.g. unaffected family members). They can be used to facilitate diagnosis and in the search for causative genes in addiction disorders.

1.2 Stages of addiction

Addiction does not develop immediately. Rather, its development should be thought of as a process made up of several stages that are composed of elements (see Figure 1.1). Upon the initialization of substance use, the individual may pursue some course of action for appetitive effects or motives (e.g. pain reduction, affect enhancement, arousal manipulation). There has been a clustering of different addictive behaviours, involving hedonistic (e.g. drug use, sex, gambling) or nurturant (e.g. shopping addiction, love, exercise) motives. Other or additional motives may be plausible, however (e.g. to achieve fantasy or oblivion). All addictions may have in common the capacity to alter the subjective experience of the self.

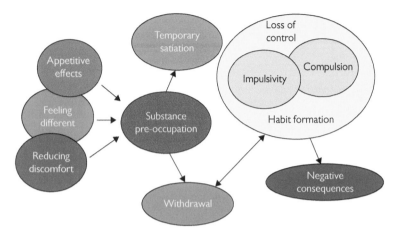

Figure 1.1 **Stages of addiction.** Illustration of the proposed stages of addiction and their elements.

Addiction unfolds within some individuals but not others. This may be a reflection of individual differences prior to engaging in substance use. Many self-described addicts, for example, have reported feeling 'different' from others prior to developing an addiction. These differences have been described to include feeling relatively uncomfortable, lonely, restless, or incomplete. Once a behaviour is tried (e.g. drinking alcohol) that decreases or eliminates the reference point of discomfort, a process of addiction may unfold. This explains why pre-existing psychopathologies (e.g. anxiety, depression) may be a trigger for the emergence of substance use in some individuals. This pre-existing vulnerability may also be genetic in origin, accounting for up to 50% of the variance of addiction.

Many people, however, do not report **feeling different** prior to developing an addiction. Instead, these individuals may engage in substance use as it is perceived as highly valued or enjoyable. This inflated evaluation may possibly come from the rapid effects that occur from substance use and which the person desires to repeat. The initial reaction to substance use may be experienced as extremely positive, making it particularly appealing. This is not to say, however, that in these individuals, there is no pre-existing propensity (e.g. trait impulsivity, sensation seeking) that influences them to engage in substance use.

The **preoccupation** with substance use may begin to develop following the initial appetitive effects. This second aspect of addiction involves excessive thoughts about the substance and excessive time spent planning to use the substance. Here, behaviour related to substance use 'spills over' into several aspects of a person's daily life. Less time is spent on other activities despite the potentially diminishing appetitive effects of the substance.

Tolerance and withdrawal are physiological hallmarks of addiction that contribute to preoccupation. Tolerance is seen as a need to engage in substance use at a relatively greater level in order to achieve the same desired effects. As tolerance increases, the person needs more alcohol or other drugs. This will lead to spending more time locating and engaging in substance use. This indicates an increasing preoccupation.

Withdrawal refers to physiological or acquired discomfort experienced upon the abrupt termination of the substance. If withdrawal symptoms exist and worsen, a person is likely to spend greater amounts of time recovering from after-effects (e.g. hangovers). Thus, the processes of tolerance and withdrawal will mean the person spends more time locating, engaging, and recovering from substance use. For many addicts, the initial period of substance use is driven by pleasure. Over time, the motivation to use switches to a desire to minimize withdrawal.

Also possibly related to tolerance or withdrawal is **craving**. Craving (i.e. urges) to engage in substance use has become a defining feature of addiction. Craving is not the same thing as physiological withdrawal. Instead, it involves an intense urge to engage in a specific act and may be experienced long after the dissipation of withdrawal. Craving is often a precipitator of relapse and is now a target for the development of relapse prevention medications. Craving has also been proposed as a diagnostic feature of the addictions to be added to the DSM-V.

Temporary **satiation**, experienced during acute engagement in the addictive behaviour, is also experienced during the process of addiction. This has been described by addicts as a sense of distraction from life's problems. Here, acute substance use becomes increasingly more incentivized (i.e. gains greater incentive value). Non-addictive alternatives may lose incentive value over time despite the discomfort in trying to achieve satiation. There are instances, however, in which the person suffering from addiction reports no longer being able to achieve satiation from substance use, presumably due to excessive tolerance.

Drug addiction is characterized by continued use and recurrent relapse despite serious negative consequences. Addicts often report feeling compelled towards substance use while sensing incomplete control over their behaviour. This appears to implicate decrements in higher order cognitive functioning, akin to a **loss of control**.

Impulsiveness has been suggested to indicate an addiction-related loss of control. This may involve spontaneous urges to engage in substance use. Loss of control may further suggest a struggle between implicit (unconscious) and declarative (conscious) systems. The implicit system may facilitate impulsive behaviour associated with addiction related events, which are strongly embedded in memory. The declarative system, in turn, may fail to inhibit automatic (i.e. unconscious) substance use in response to craving.

This suggests that a loss of control during addiction involves competing neural signals between primitive, reflexive brain regions that kindle impulsivity and higher brain areas that involve cognitive processing (e.g. behavioural inhibition). Indeed, research is beginning to elucidate why a loss of cognitive control may be a central component for both the initiation of, and continued, substance abuse (see Chapter 4).

1.3 Conclusion

Negative consequences (e.g. physical discomfort, social disapproval, financial loss, or decreased self-esteem) will begin to take hold following chronic substance use. Indeed, continuing to engage in the addictive behaviour, despite suffering numerous negative consequences, is a criterion for dependence. There may also be a fear of having to cope with the perceived day-to-day stresses of life upon substance use cessation. This may be due to an accumulation of addiction-related consequences (e.g. debts) or having to endure raw emotional experiences without concurrent self-medication.

The failure to learn to cope without substance use and suffering withdrawal-related phenomena may additionally add to this element of negativity. Negative consequences may vary across contexts. However, role consequences (e.g. difficulty fulfilling one's role as parent, spouse, or co-worker) are usual aspects of this negativity. Importantly, such negative consequences may bring **negative reinforcement**. Here, substance-dependent individuals are likely to further engage in substance use in order to eliminate or reduce the physical and psychological discomfort experienced as a result of chronic addiction behaviour.

REFERENCES

American Psychiatric Association (2013). *Diagnostic and Statistical Manual of Mental Disorders.* 5th edition. Washington, DC: American Psychiatric Press.

Dalley JW, Fryer TD, Brichard L, et al. (2007). Nucleus accumbens D2/3 receptors predict trait impulsivity and cocaine reinforcement. *Science,* **315**, 1267–70.

Ersche KD, Turton AJ, Pradhan S, et al. (2010). Drug addiction endophenotypes: impulsive versus sensation-seeking personality traits. *Biological Psychiatry,* **68**, 770–3.

Goodman A (1990). Addiction: definition and implications. *British Journal of Addiction,* **85**, 1403–8.

Gould RW, Duke AN, and Nader MA (2013). PET studies in non-human primate models of cocaine abuse: translational research related to vulnerability and neuroadaptations. *Neuropharmacology,* **pii**, S0028–3908(13)00046–44.

Meyer RE (1996). The disease called addiction: emerging evidence in a 200-year debate. *Lancet,* **347**, 162–6.

Sussman S and Sussman AN (2011). Considering the definition of addiction. *International Journal of Environmental Research and Public Health,* **8**, 4025–38.

World Health Organization (1992). The ICD-10 classification of mental and behavioural disorders: clinical descriptions and diagnostic guidelines. Geneva: World Health Organization.

CHAPTER 2

Burden of addiction

KEY POINTS

- Tobacco use is still the leading cause of preventable death in the world.
- Alcohol use is associated with massive and growing global disability, particularly in young males.
- Drug-related deaths are steadily increasing.
- The vast majority of global substance-related problems are in men.
- Substance addiction confers social/psychological/physical burdens on the individual.
- Substance addiction confers significant costs to society.

Substances of abuse (e.g. alcohol, cocaine, heroin, tobacco) are major causes of harm to individuals and society. Because of the harm some of these substances cause, they are scheduled under the United Nations 1961 Single Convention on Narcotic Drugs and the 1971 Convention on Psychotropic Substances.

This chapter will address the scale and cost of substance abuse to society. These costs to society are on a number of levels, most significantly to those whose health is adversely compromised by substance abuse and addiction.

2.1 Tobacco

While tobacco use is not associated with significant psychological and social impairment synonymous with substance abuse and addiction, it is the leading cause of preventable death in the world. Nicotine is the main addictive component in cigarettes leading to addiction, which can have significant medical consequences, and the cessation of smoking is a critical prerequisite to improving health (e.g. cancer recovery, cardiovascular rehabilitation). Tobacco use is a significant risk factor for premature death, associated with the eight leading causes of death in the world (see Figure 2.1). Therefore, tobacco addiction still remains a major obstacle with respect to increasing the longevity of health and reducing the burden of tobacco-related diseases in populations across the world.

Figure 2.1 **Tobacco use and premature death.** Hatched areas indicate proportions of deaths that are related to tobacco use and are coloured according to the column of the respective cause of death.

Reprinted from *WHO Report on the Global Tobacco Epidemic*, The MPOWER package. Copyright (2008) World Health Organization.

2.2 Young people

Young people, aged 10–24 years, represent ~27% of the world's population. The health of young people, however, is largely neglected in global public health debate due to the perception that young people are healthy by virtue of their age. Compared to adults, however, people in adolescence are more likely to exhibit a number of psychological traits, such as risky and reward-seeking behaviour, that increase the potential likelihood of substance misuse and addiction. Research shows that substance misuse is one of the main causes of **global** disability in young (15–24-year-old) people (see Figure 2.2)—particularly involving the use of alcohol in males.

2.3 Brain disorders

Disorders of the brain, particularly mental disorders, contribute 26.6% of the total cause of burden in the European Union. These disorders are the largest contributor to all-cause morbidity burden, as measured by disability-adjusted life-years (DALYs). DALYs are defined as the sum of years of potential life lost due to premature mortality and the years of productive life lost due to disability. Significantly, alcohol use disorders have been found to be among the top four most disabling single conditions, as measured by DALYs (see Figure 2.3). Furthermore, drug use disorders are also amongst the most frequent.

Figure 2.2 Alcohol and global disability in young people. DALYs attributable to the most important risk factors by region and sex in 2004 in 15–24 year-olds. DALY = disability-adjusted life-year. Physical injuries refer to unintentional injuries resulting from occupational risks.

Reprinted from *The Lancet*, 377, Gore, F. M., Bloem, P. J., Patton, G. C., et al. Global burden of disease in young people aged 10–24 years: a systematic analysis. pp. 2093–2102. Copyright (2011), with permission from Elsevier.

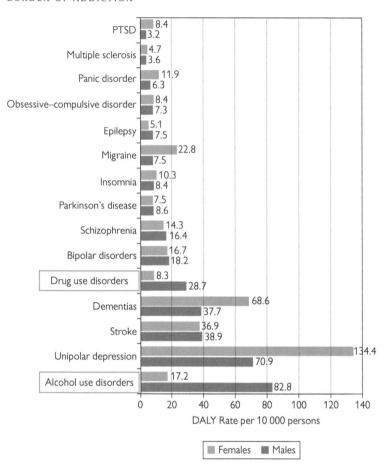

Figure 2.3 Alcohol use as a disabling brain condition. The size and burden of mental disorders and other disorders of the brain in Europe 2010. This study shows that alcohol was one of the four most disabling single conditions, along with depression, dementias, and stroke. Drug use disorders were also prevalent.

Reprinted from *European Neuropsychopharmacology*, 21, Wittchen, H. U., Jacobi, F., Rehm, J., et al. The size and burden of mental disorders and other disorders of the brain in Europe 2010, pp. 655–679, Copyright (2011), with permission from Elsevier.

2.4 Alcohol

Despite the majority of the world's adult population abstaining from alcohol, almost 50% of adults consume alcohol in any given year. This pattern and level of alcohol consumption is potentially problematic—high volumes of alcohol are being consumed, particularly during heavy drinking sessions (i.e. binges). This pattern of alcohol use is leading to premature mortality and, equally, a burden of disease and injury to societies where this level of alcohol use is occurring.

Deaths attributable to alcohol on a global scale, for example, appear to be higher in men, with the highest rates observed in Europe (see Figure 2.4). Globally, the burden of disease attributable to alcohol is also higher in males, which appears to be at its highest in Europe (see Figure 2.5). Furthermore, the prevalence of alcohol-use disorders is higher in men (see Figure 2.6).

2.5 Policy

The control of substances in the United Kingdom is represented by domestic legislation—the 1971 Misuse of Drugs Act (as amended). Substances, most notably alcohol and tobacco, are regulated by taxation, sales, and restrictions on the age of purchase. Newly available substances, such as mephedrone (4-methylmethcathinone), have recently been made illegal in the United Kingdom

	AFR	AMR	EMR	EUR	SEAR	WPR	World	World 2000
Men	3.7%	9.0%	0.8%	11.0%	3.9%	8.4%	6.3%	5.6%
Women	1.0%	1.8%	0.1%	1.8%	0.5%	1.5%	1.1%	0.6%
Both	2.4%	5.6%	0.5%	6.5%	2.3%	5.3%	3.8%	3.2%

Figure 2.4 Deaths attributable to alcohol higher in men globally. Alcohol-attributable deaths as a proportion of all deaths by sex and WHO region in 2004. AFR = African region. AMR = American region. EMR = eastern Mediterranean region. EUR = European region. SEAR = South East Asian region. WPR = western Pacific region.

Reprinted from *The Lancet*, 373, Rehm, J., Mathers, C., Popova, S., et al. Global burden of disease and injury and economic cost attributable to alcohol use and alcohol-use disorders, pp. 2223–2233. Copyright (2009), with permission from Elsevier.

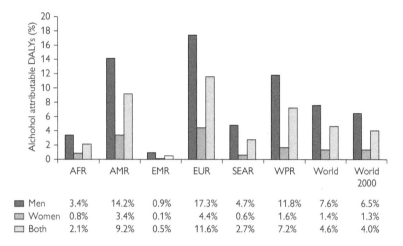

Figure 2.5 Burden of disease attributable to alcohol is higher in men. Alcohol-attributable burden of disease in disability-adjusted life-years (DALYs) as a proportion of all DALYs by sex and WHO region in 2004. AFR = African region. AMR = American region. EMR = eastern Mediterranean region. EUR = European region. SEAR = South East Asian region. WPR = western Pacific region.

Reprinted from *The Lancet*, 373, Rehm, J., Mathers, C., Popova, S., et al. Global burden of disease and injury and economic cost attributable to alcohol use and alcohol-use disorders, pp. 2223–2233. Copyright (2009), with permission from Elsevier.

on the basis of concerns about their harms while the law on other substances, particularly cannabis, has been toughened due to similar concerns regarding their potential detriment to mental health (e.g. onset of psychosis in adolescence).

While there is considerable social concern regarding the health and social consequences of harder, more illicit drug use (e.g. crack cocaine, heroin), there appears to be overwhelming evidence that alcohol use is still a major cause for concern. In a recent study conducted by the Independent Scientific Committee on Drugs, the 20 most frequently used drugs were scored on 16 criteria: 9 related to the harms that a drug produces in the individual and 7 to the harms drugs cause to others. Drugs were scored out of 100 points and the criteria were weighted to indicate their relative importance. The research reported that the most harmful drugs to users were heroin and crack cocaine whereas the most harmful to others was alcohol. It was also shown that when the two part-scores were combined, alcohol was the **most** harmful, followed by heroin and crack cocaine (see Figure 2.7).

While the current use of illicit drugs in the United Kingdom has been declining since the 1990s, the number of recorded drug-related deaths between 1996 and 2010 actually increased by 67.5%. In 2010, there were 1,930 drug-related deaths,

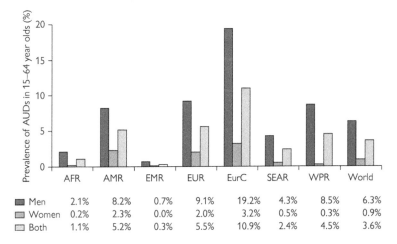

	AFR	AMR	EMR	EUR	EurC	SEAR	WPR	World
Men	2.1%	8.2%	0.7%	9.1%	19.2%	4.3%	8.5%	6.3%
Women	0.2%	2.3%	0.0%	2.0%	3.2%	0.5%	0.3%	0.9%
Both	1.1%	5.2%	0.3%	5.5%	10.9%	2.4%	4.5%	3.6%

Figure 2.6 **One-year prevalence of alcohol-use disorders (AUDs) in people aged 15–64 years by sex and WHO region in 2004. AFR = African region. AMR = American region. EMR = eastern Mediterranean region. EUR = European region. EurC = eastern European region with proportionally higher adult mortality than other European parts (most populous country: Russia). SEAR = South East Asian region. WPR = western Pacific region.**

Reprinted from *The Lancet*, 373, Rehm, J., Mathers, C., Popova, S., et al. Global burden of disease and injury and economic cost attributable to alcohol use and alcohol-use disorders, pp. 2223–2233. Copyright (2009), with permission from Elsevier.

equivalent to a rate of 3.10 per 100,000/population (all ages). The vast majority of these were among men (79.4%), and the rate was highest in the 35 to 39 years' age group.

Most of the drug-related deaths in the United Kingdom continue to be linked to the use of opioid drugs—primarily heroin/morphine and methadone, followed by cocaine and ecstasy (see Table 2.1). Overdoses related to opioid use are predominantly caused by respiratory depression while cocaine-related deaths usually result from myocardial infarction or stroke. Ecstasy-related deaths result from hyperthermia or hyponatraemia. It is perhaps worth noting that some categories of illicit drugs, including cannabis, present no risk of death by overdose.

The increased risk of death from drug overdose is associated with poverty, homelessness, and polysubstance use, impaired physical health, depression, and a previous history of drug overdose. Illicit drug users are also known to have higher rates of completed and attempted suicide compared to the general population. This is associated with psychopathology, family dysfunction, social isolation, and polydrug use.

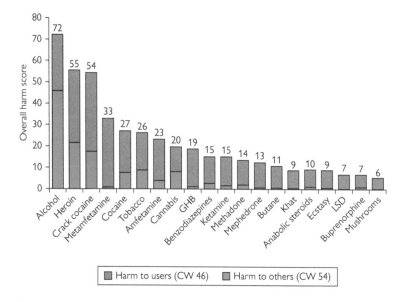

Figure 2.7 Alcohol tops drug harms to others in the United Kingdom. Drugs ordered by their overall harm scores, showing the separate contributions to the overall scores of harms to users and harm to others. The weights after normalization (0–100) are shown in the key (cumulative in the sense of the sum of all the normalized weights for all the criteria to users, 46; and for all the criteria to others, 54). CW = cumulative weight. GHB = γ-hydroxybutyric acid. LSD = lysergic acid diethylamide.

Reprinted from *The Lancet*, 376, Nutt, D. J., King, L. A., & Phillips, L. D., Drug harms in the UK: a multicriteria decision analysis, pp. 1558–1565. Copyright (2010), with permission from Elsevier.

2.6 Conclusion

Estimates for the cost of substance use to society in economic terms are limited. These include costs to the individual, such as the costs related to premature death, drug-related illness, and the loss of earnings through criminality/imprisonment, sickness, temporary or permanent unemployment, and reduced educational attainment. The costs to society can usually be divided into four broad categories:

Healthcare service costs—this includes costs to primary care and hospital services (A&E, medical and surgical inpatient services, paediatric services, psychiatric services, and outpatient departments).

Costs of drug-related crime, disorder, and antisocial behaviour—including costs to the criminal justice system, costs to services (e.g. social

Table 2.1 Drug mentions on death certificates in the UK, 2002–10.

Drug	Year									
	2002	2003	2004	2005	2006	2007	2008	2009	2010	% change 2002–10
Heroin	1118	883	977	1043	985	1130	1243	1210	1061	–5.1
Methadone	300	292	300	292	339	441	565	582	503	67.6
Cocaine	161	161	192	221	224	246	325	238	180	11.8
Ecstasy	79	66	61	73	62	64	55	32	9	–88.6

Source data from Davies C, English L, Stewart C, et al. (2011). *United Kingdom drug situation: annual report to the European Monitoring Centre for Drugs and Drug Addiction (EMCDDA) 2011*. United Kingdom Focal Point at the Department of Health, London.

work services), costs of drunk-/drug-driving, and the human cost of substance-related harm (e.g. domestic abuse, assault).

Loss of productivity and profitability in the workplace—this includes costs to the economy from substance-related deaths and substance-related lost working days.

Impact on family and social networks—including human and emotional costs, such as breakdown of marital and family relationships, poverty, loss of employment, domestic and child abuse, and homelessness.

FURTHER READING

Davies C, English L, Stewart C, et al. (2011). *United Kingdom drug situation: annual report to the European Monitoring Centre for Drugs and Drug Addiction (EMCDDA) 2011*. London: United Kingdom Focal Point at the Department of Health.

Ellison RC (ed.) (2007). Health risks and benefits of moderate alcohol consumption: proceedings of an international symposium. *Annals of Epidemiology*, **17** (Suppl.), S1–S116.

Gore FM, Bloem PJ, Patton GC, et al. (2011). Global burden of disease in young people aged 10–24 years: a systematic analysis. *Lancet*, **377**, 2093–102.

Grant M and Litvak J (eds) (1998). *Drinking Patterns and their Consequences*. Washington, DC: Taylor & Francis.

Nutt DJ, King LA, and Phillips LD (2010). Drug harms in the UK: a multicriteria decision analysis. *Lancet*, **376**, 1558–65.

Rehm J, Mathers C, Popova S, et al. (2009). Global burden of disease and injury and economic cost attributable to alcohol use and alcohol-use disorders. *Lancet*, **373**, 2223–33.

Stimson GV, Grant M, Choquet M, et al. (eds) (2007). *Drinking in Context: Patterns, Interventions, and Partnerships*. New York, NY: Routledge.

Wittchen HU, Jacobi F, Rehm J, et al. (2011). The size and burden of mental disorders and other disorders of the brain in Europe 2010. *European Neuropsychopharmacology*, **21**, 655–79.

CHAPTER 2

Key elements of addiction

- Addictive substances are highly reinforcing.
- They are reinforcing because they induce pleasure.
- Pleasure leads to 'liking' the effects of addictive substances.
- 'Liking' a substance can become conditioned to substance-related cues.
- 'Wanting' a substance can occur at the expense of 'liking' the substance.
- Excessive 'wanting' can lead to a loss of control of substance use.
- Substance use habits are unconscious—they are automatic.
- Withdrawal from substances of abuse leads to repeated use.
- Craving for substances may occur following prolonged abstinence.
- Craving may trigger substance relapse.

Addiction is characterized by the compulsion to seek and take a substance (or engage in behaviours, such as gambling), the loss of control in limiting substance intake, and the emergence of a negative emotional state (e.g. dysphoria, anxiety) when substance intake is prevented (see Figure 3.1). Elements of addiction during the addiction trajectory are a reflection of changes in brain homeostasis. These homeostatic changes ultimately lead to: (1) a decreased sensitivity for natural rewards; (2) an enhanced sensitivity for conditioned substance cues and the expectation of substance use rewards; (3) a weakened control over substance use urges and substance-taking behaviour; and (4) substance tolerance and withdrawal.

3.1 Key elements of addiction

3.1.1 Liking

Whatever the initial reason for substance use in individuals (e.g. reducing discomfort, sensation seeking), substances of abuse are highly positively reinforcing (i.e. rewarding). They are rewarding, particularly during the initial phases of use, because they induce a conscious experience of pleasure.

This pleasure induces 'liking'. 'Liking' is related to activity in discrete hedonic 'hot spots' within the reward circuitry of the brain (see Chapter 4). Activity in these 'hot spots' has been shown to be increased in animals, together with 'liking' reactions, when they are stimulated. Unconscious (or implicit) 'liking' reactions to hedonic stimuli are also possible without the conscious feelings of pleasure.

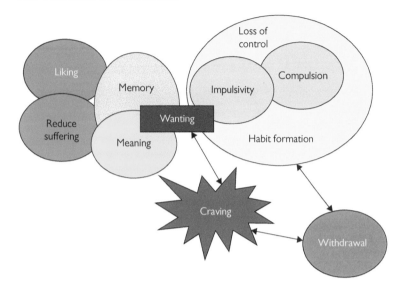

Figure 3.1 **The key elements of addiction.**

The enhancement of 'liking', however, is both restricted and fragile. These 'liking' systems are relatively inflexible to activation compared to 'wanting' systems (see 3.1.5 Wanting).

This 'liking' of substance-induced pleasure may, in some individuals, lead to an inflated evaluation of the substance. This exaggerated appraisal of pleasure is likely to positively reinforce the desire to repeat substance use. Similarly, the initial response to a substance that is not liked by an individual, but rather appraised as aversive (i.e. disliked), will be negatively reinforced—the individual will not continue to use (though tobacco is an exception because users have to overcome the unpleasantness of the initial smoking experience in order to benefit from the effects).

As substance use increases, reinforcement can become more pronounced in response to cues associated with the substance (e.g. people, objects, places). These responses to cues can be greater than that produced by the substance itself. Therefore, the 'liking' of the pleasurable effects of substances during the initial stages of use is accompanied by the formation of powerful conditioned responses to the substance—cues can trigger the expectation of ensuing pleasure.

Responses to substance cues have also been shown to correlate with the subjective experience of craving in substance dependence. This associative learning, therefore, drives the incessant preoccupation with, and craving of, the substance. This can provoke relapse during abstinence.

3.1.2 Reducing suffering

Many people turn to substance use in order to reduce pain—either physical or psychological—in a form of self-medication. The use of alcohol, for example, to reduce performance anxiety or social anxiety disorder is a form of self-medicating. Social anxiety disorder is a very common disorder and is the most common diagnosable disorder in alcoholism—a quarter of young male alcoholics suffer from this disorder. Other populations find that different drugs can help with their underlying condition. People with ADHD (attention deficit hyperactive disorder), for example, find that stimulants (e.g. amphetamine) can be helpful. This population often report, following the self-administration of stimulants, that they become more calm, focused, and less distracted.

Understanding the reasons for drug use is critically important in devising the right treatment for each individual. Patients with social anxiety can respond very well to selective serotonin reuptake inhibitors (SSRIs) whereas those with ADHD require stimulants or atomoxetine. In both these groups, appropriate medical prescribing will reduce their maladaptive alcohol/drug use.

The use of opiates (e.g. morphine) in pain control is often accompanied by fears of becoming addicted. Whilst this can happen, it is relatively rare and, in most countries, there is a relative under-treatment of pain with these types of drugs because doctors fear the patient may become addicted.

3.1.3 Meaning

Some substance users explicitly state that they are only fully 'real' when under the influence of the substance. Terms, such as 'it was the missing piece of the jigsaw' or 'I felt normal for the first time when I first drank', suggest that substance use may induce a false sense of psychological security. Such experiences are particularly common in opiate and alcohol addiction and may reflect an underlying genetic propensity or some psychological problem. Nevertheless, the meaning behind substance use makes it difficult for such people to give up, as they never feel fully complete in the absence of the substance.

3.1.4 Memory

Substance addiction is a form of long-term memory—particularly for the stimuli associated with the effects of the substance. This issue of conditioned substance use memories is dealt with in Chapter 4.

3.1.5 Wanting

Substance-induced rewards that a person likes are rewards that the person wants. With repeated and excessive substance use comes an adaptive dampening down of the initial appetitive effects. It is at this point that the development of 'wanting', at the expense of pleasure and 'liking', begins to emerge. Significantly, the 'liking' and 'wanting' of rewards are dissociable, both psychologically and biologically. Wanting refers to an **incentive salience**—a type of incentive motivation that promotes approach towards, and the consumption of, rewards. In the case of substance abuse and addiction, excessive incentive salience may cause **irrational wanting** due to substance-related cues acquiring increased incentive-motivational value.

This 'wanting' for the substance, without 'liking' it, is caused by continued and excessive associative learning and a decreased sensitivity of the brain's reward circuitry to the pleasure-inducing properties of the substance itself. At this point, substances may no longer be liked but rather become compulsively wanted by the user. Importantly, brain regions for 'wanting' are more ubiquitous and more easily activated than those for 'liking'. 'Wanting' mechanisms are more numerous and diverse, which may explain the disproportionate 'wanting' of a substance reward without equally liking the same reward.

3.1.6 Craving

Preoccupation/anticipation or craving in addiction is thought to be a key element of relapse in humans. Research suggests that craving involves complex interactions between numerous neurotransmitter systems in the brain (e.g. dopamine and glutamate). Significantly, craving is not exclusive to the stage of acute substance withdrawal and, indeed, may overcome individuals who are in a protracted period of alcohol or drug abstinence. Craving may be triggered by environmental cues associated with the pleasurable effects of substances—cues that trigger conditioned memories of substance rewards. This may lead to wanting the substance and, consequently, relapse. Craving, however, has proved to be a difficult construct to measure clinically and often does not correlate well with relapse.

3.1.7 Habit

Substance addiction is characterized by a discrepancy between the user's expressed intentions to abstain from the substance and their behaviour, which is characterized by repeated relapses and continued use of the substance. The concept of 'motivational conflict' appears fundamental to understanding substance abuse and addiction. Motivational problems involving conflict between inclinations to use ('approach') and refrain from ('avoidance') the substance are highly relevant to breaking habits that are complicit in sustaining addiction.

There is evidence that substance use habits begin to originate outside of consciousness (i.e. users are unaware). The compulsive sequence of substance use behaviours become so practised that they can be extremely difficult to avoid initiating by the user. The role of implicit (or automatic) cognitive processes in substance use and addiction, where habit occurs outside the realms of consciousness, may be important to treating substance addiction. Automatic cognitive processes related to habit are spontaneous and fast, as opposed to 'controlled' cognitive processes, which are deliberate, slow, and require conscious awareness. It has been proposed that substance use leads to the development of automatic processes that promote approach behaviour towards substance-related cues and, ultimately, substance use.

Significantly, treatment strategies, during which 'controlled' processes are engaged in, either to inhibit or override these automatic approach tendencies, are likely to promote substance avoidance. Therefore, during the emergence of increased substance addiction, an approach-avoidance conflict between such automatic appetitive responses to substance cues and controlled processes will emerge. The emergence of this conflict is thought to exacerbate the preoccupation with substance use in an attempt to bring about its resolution as well as lead to secondary psychiatric issues, such as anxiety and depression.

3.1.8 Withdrawal

For many addicts, the initial period of drug use is driven by pleasure. Over time, the motivation to use switches to a desire to minimize withdrawal. Withdrawal usually refers to physiological symptoms experienced upon the abrupt termination of the substance. The response that follows the stage of drug intoxication differs markedly across drugs and is influenced by the chronicity and frequency of its abuse. For some drugs, such as opiates, alcohol, and sedative hypnotics, drug discontinuation in chronic users can trigger an intense, acute physical withdrawal syndrome. If not properly managed, a severe physical withdrawal syndrome can sometimes be fatal.

All drugs of abuse are associated with a motivational withdrawal syndrome characterized by dysphoria, irritability, emotional distress, and sleep disturbances. These symptoms can persist, even after protracted withdrawal.

3.2 Conclusion

Acute withdrawal is distinct from protracted or motivational withdrawal, but both contribute to relapse. Both the physical and psychological withdrawal symptoms during acute abstinence involve a process of attempting to achieve a new state of stability (i.e. homeostasis) within endogenous systems responsible for maintaining the internal stability of the organism. Relapse during withdrawal may be a form of negative reinforcement—using substances to minimize the unpleasantness of withdrawal.

FURTHER READING

Barkby H, Dickson JM, Roper L, et al. (2011). To approach or avoid alcohol? Automatic and self-reported motivational tendencies in alcohol dependence. *Alcoholism: Clinical and Experimental Research*, **36**, 361–8.

Berridge KC, Robinson TE, and Aldridge JW (2009). Dissecting components of reward: 'liking', 'wanting', and learning. *Current Opinion in Pharmacology*, **9**, 65–73.

Christiansen P, Cole JC, Goudie AJ, et al. (2012). Components of behavioural impulsivity and automatic cue approach predict unique variance in hazardous drinking. *Psychopharmacology (Berl)*, **219**, 501–10.

Goldstein RZ, Woicik PA, Moeller SJ, et al. (2010). Liking and wanting of drug and non-drug rewards in active cocaine users: the STRAP-R questionnaire. *Journal of Psychopharmacology*, **24**, 257–66.

Koob GF and Volkow ND (2010). Neurocircuitry of addiction. *Neuropsychopharmacology*, **35**, 217–38.

Zorick T, Nestor L, Miotto K, et al. (2010). Withdrawal symptoms in abstinent methamphetamine-dependent subjects. *Addiction*, **105**, 1809–18.

CHAPTER 3

Neurobiological processes in addiction

- The brain controls necessary motivational and cognitive processes.
- These processes involve a network of independent and overlapping brain circuits.
- These processes involve reward, motivation, learning/memory, and cognition.
- Reward involves dopamine in the ventral striatum.
- Learning involves dopamine in the ventral tegmental area and ventral striatum.
- Memory involves glutamate in the amygdala and hippocampus.
- Motivation and drive involve GABA and dopamine in the orbitofrontal cortex.
- Cognition involves dopamine and glutamate in the prefrontal cortex.
- These processes are disrupted by substances of addiction.

There are a number of regions in the brain involved in controlling necessary motivational and cognitive processes. These processes can be disrupted by substances of addiction. The key neural substrates underlying these processes are made up of a network of four independent and overlapping circuits (see Figure 4.1).

We will discuss the neural substrates underlying the control of these motivational and cognitive processes and consider the potential implications of their disruption by substances of addiction.

4.1 Reward

Reward is a central component for driving incentive-based learning, eliciting appropriate responses to stimuli, and the development of goal-directed behaviours. Knowledge regarding reward regions came from research in rodents by Olds and Milner. They revealed that rats would work vigorously to obtain electrical stimulation of multiple areas of the brain that form part of a reward circuit.

The core component of this reward-related circuitry is the nucleus accumbens (NAcc) in the ventral striatum (VS). The VS receives input from dopamine cell bodies in the ventral tegmental area (VTA) of the midbrain via the mesolimbic pathway. Dopamine neurons of the nigrostriatal pathway project from the substantia nigra to the dorsal striatum (caudate nucleus). In rats, electrical stimulation of a pathway, known as the medial forebrain bundle, is highly rewarding.

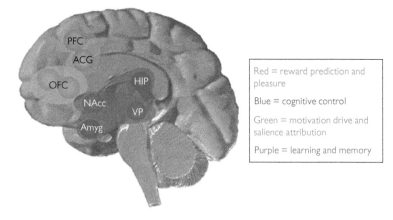

Figure 4.1 Key neural substrates. The network of four independent and overlapping circuits consisting of: (i) reward (in red), located within the nucleus accumbens (NAcc)/ventral striatum (VS) and ventral pallidum (VP); (ii) motivation and/or drive (in green), located in the orbitofrontal cortex (OFC); (iii) learning and memory (in purple), located in the amygdala (Amyg) and hippocampus (HIP); and (iv) cognitive control (in blue), located in the prefrontal cortex (PFC) and cingulate gyrus (ACG).

Reprinted from *Trends in Molecular Medicine*, 12, Baler, R. D. & Volkow, N. D., Drug addiction: the neurobiology of disrupted self-control, pp. 559–566, Copyright (2006), with permission from Elsevier.

This nerve pathway links the VTA with the NAcc/VS. Rodents also learn to self-administer amphetamine, cocaine, or dopamine receptor agonists directly into the VS. This suggests that increased dopamine transmission in the VS is involved in reward.

The firing of dopamine VTA neurons in response to reward involves phasic (i.e. fast) short-burst firing. VTA dopamine neurons also provide a predictive signal about rewards. Dopamine released from VTA neurons binds with dopamine D1 and D2 receptors (D1/2R) in the VS. Binding to the D1R increases the excitability of neurons. Binding to DR2 decreases excitability. Dopamine binding to D2R is generally thought to encode information related to expected reward value and the reward itself.

A number of other neurotransmitter systems influence VS reward circuitry. Inhibitory gamma-aminobutyric acid (GABA) neurons are located in the VS. GABA neurons project from the NAcc to the ventral pallidum (VP) via the striato-pallidal pathway. Glutamate is an excitatory neurotransmitter. Glutamate projections from the PFC to the VS are important for learning about rewards (see 4.3 Learning and memory). Additional key substrates of this reward circuitry are also targets of dopamine projections from the VTA. These include the amygdala

(Amyg), hippocampus (HIP), orbitofrontal cortex (OFC), anterior cingulate gyrus (ACG), and prefrontal cortex (PFC).

Substances of addiction (e.g. alcohol, stimulants) are highly rewarding. They are rewarding because they induce a conscious experience of pleasure. This pleasure leads to 'liking' (see Chapter 3). Pre-clinical research has shown that there are discrete hedonic 'hot spots' for this 'liking'. Specifically, a region within the outer (shell) portion of the NAcc and a region within the posterior VP elicit 'liking' responses. Rats learn to self-administer dopaminergic drugs (e.g. cocaine, D1R/D2R receptor agonists) more into the shell of the NAcc than the core. Opioid, endocannabinoid, and GABA-benzodiazepine neurotransmitter systems also appear to be important for generating many pleasurable, 'liking' reactions to rewards.

All substances of addiction work by triggering transient, exaggerated increases in VS dopamine. These surges in dopamine release resemble and can, in the case of stimulants (e.g. cocaine, amphetamine), greatly surpass the physiological increases triggered by natural rewards (e.g. food, water). Research is beginning to show that the progression from initial substance use to addiction involves synaptic plasticity (i.e. the strengthening of connections between neurons) in this VS reward pathway. This suggests that the hard-wired circuitry essential for the processing of natural rewards can be unfavourably commandeered by substances of abuse.

Importantly, the release of dopamine at the VS is not necessary for all forms of reward learning and 'liking'. It may involve just the 'wanting' of a reward (see Chapter 3). 'Wanting' in the absence of 'liking' is a critical characteristic of addiction. Increased 'wanting' involves a disproportional change in the motivational value of substance rewards.

4.2 Motivation and drive

Rewards are motivating because they are reinforcing—they are actively sought out and approached by animals and humans. Motivation and drive are important elements for the survival of the species. They involve a vigorous goal-directed pursuit of rewards. Goal-directed behaviour involves the integration and processing of information about multiple changing internal states and environmental conditions.

The initiation and organization of motivated behaviour depends on the dopamine system. Projections from the VTA to VS are, in part, responsible for initiating the motivation for rewards. The NAcc portion serves as a critical interface between limbic and motor systems—linking motivation with action. The VTA-NAcc dopamine pathway is thought to be part of a gating mechanism. This mechanism directs the translation of motive states into motor responses.

The OFC is also involved in the processes of motivation and drive for rewards. The OFC is located on the ventral surface of the PFC. It is connected with brain regions involved in dopamine-dependent reinforcement. The NAcc projects to the OFC, and the OFC also receives direct dopamine projections from the VTA. OFC functioning appears to be particularly important for guiding goal-directed behaviour for rewards. In healthy individuals, there is increased activation in the OFC during actual decision-making for rewards and the evaluation of reward outcomes. The OFC is also involved in the attribution of salience to reinforcing stimuli.

The development of irrational 'wanting' of substance rewards, at the expense of 'liking' them, emerges as addiction develops (i.e. there is increased incentive salience for substance rewards). The enhanced motivation to procure substances becomes a hallmark of addiction. This is often triggered by substance-related cues (i.e. stimuli associated with the substance). Substance abusers show hyperactivity in the OFC during cue-induced craving. During protracted withdrawal, substance abusers demonstrate hypoactivity in the OFC.

Following chronic substance use, dysfunction of the **striato-thalamo-orbitofrontal circuit** is thought to inappropriately intensify the motivation to procure and self-administer substances. Through its connections with the NAcc/VS, the OFC may learn to overattribute salience to substance rewards and cues. OFC activity in response to cues associated with highly incentivized substance rewards may also override OFC activity necessary for optimal decision-making. This has important implications for abstinence. Excessive substance 'wanting' and sub-optimal decision-making are likely to trigger relapse in response to substance-related cues.

4.3 Learning and memory

The linking of motivation with actions to obtain rewards must be learned and encoded in memory for future use. There is considerable evidence that dopamine is involved in learning and memory processes. The role of dopamine in the consolidation of memories also appears to be particularly important.

Dopamine release at the NAcc/VS acts as a teaching signal—it is involved in making predictions about future rewards. The dopamine response to reward delivery appears to code a **prediction error**. Rewards that are better than predicted elicit activation (i.e. positive prediction error). A fully predicted reward elicits no response. A reward that is worse than predicted induces a depression (i.e. negative prediction error). Dopamine neurons in the VS respond to reward only to the extent to which it differs from the prediction. Therefore, dopamine neurons in the VS are activated only when the current reward is **better** than the previous reward.

Much evidence for the role of dopamine-dependent neural substrates in learning and memory comes from findings in associative learning. This is the process by which an association between two stimuli (or a stimulus and behaviour) is learned. There are two forms of associative learning: **classical** and **operant**. In classical conditioning, a neutral stimulus is repeatedly paired with a reflex eliciting stimulus until the neutral stimulus elicits the same reflex response on its own. For operant conditioning, a particular behaviour is either positively (i.e. produces pleasure) or negatively (i.e. reduces discomfort) reinforced. Actions that are reinforced increase the probability that the same action will occur again in the future.

Dopamine neurons are activated upon exposure to conditioned stimuli associated with rewards. This suggests that dopamine neurons facilitate associative learning. Both the Amyg and the NAcc have been implicated in conditioned learning. Habit learning results in well-learned sequences of behaviour that are elicited automatically by appropriate stimuli (see Chapter 3). Both the caudate nucleus and putamen have been implicated in habit learning. Importantly, functional magnetic resonance imaging (fMRI) studies in humans have also pointed to the role of the striatum (i.e. caudate, putamen, NAcc/VS, VP) as well as the OFC and lateral PFC in learning. This appears consistent with the dense dopaminergic projections these regions receive from the midbrain VTA.

Since drugs of abuse increase dopamine in the VS, they will inherently facilitate the consolidation of substance use memories and experiences. Evidence points to similar physiological processes involved in both learning and memory and substance addiction: **long-term potentiation (LTP)** and **long-term depression (LTD)** involving glutamate release. LTP and LTD produce long-lasting increases and decreases, respectively, in synaptic transmission. These cellular mechanisms are thought to underlie information storage. They take place within dopamine-rich areas of the brain which are targeted by substances of abuse (e.g. VTA). These cellular mechanisms are rapidly established, maintained for long periods of time, and strengthened by repetition. Substance-induced alterations in VTA signalling can be communicated to other brain regions innervated by VTA dopamine neurons (e.g. Amyg, NAcc/VS, OFC).

Through the over-stimulation of dopamine neurons in response to the rewarding effects of substances of addiction, conditioned functional connections are established in the brain. This conditioning facilitates the consolidation of abnormal memory traces connected to the pleasure and 'liking' of substance use. Consequently, all types of substance-associated stimuli (or cues) can activate the reward circuitry associated with pleasure and 'liking'. This is due to the learned expectation of receiving the substance reward that was originally pleasurable. The recruitment of glutamate over dopamine-dependent substrates in addiction has significant implications for medications that enhance the extinction of learning in substance abuse and dependence.

4.4 Cognitive control

Cognitive control involves flexible goal-directed behaviour. This requires an adaptive cognitive control system in the brain for organizing and optimizing processing pathways. Cognitive control processes include a broad class of mental operations. These include planning, working memory (i.e. holding multiple temporary pieces of information in the mind), attention, problem-solving, response inhibition, and action monitoring. Evidence is continually emerging regarding the contributions of the PFC in the service of these cognitive control processes.

The dorsolateral prefrontal cortex (DLPFC) is located in the lateral, upper, and anterior portions of the cerebrum. The DLPFC is involved in the 'online' processing of information (i.e. working memory). This area is also involved in response inhibition, verbal fluency, set shifting, planning, organizational skills, reasoning, and problem-solving. The DLPFC receives dopamine projections from the midbrain VTA via the mesocortical pathway. Dopamine activity in the DLPFC involved in the modulation of these processes is thought to involve tonic (i.e. slow) signalling through the D1R.

The anterior cingulate gyrus (ACG) is a midline region of the brain located around the anterior portion of the corpus callosum. There is strong evidence that the ACG consists of two major subdivisions which have distinct functions. These consist of the dorsal-cognitive and rostral-ventral affective divisions. Various functions have been ascribed to the dorsal-cognitive division. These functions include the monitoring of competition between stimuli, complex motor control, error detection, working memory, and the anticipation of cognitive demand. The ACG also receives dopamine projections from the midbrain VTA via the mesocortical pathway.

In addition to its role in motivation and drive (described in 4.2 Motivation and drive), the OFC plays a key role in cognitive control processes. As part of the ventrolateral PFC (VLPFC), it is involved in impulse control and monitoring ongoing behaviour. The VLPFC plays a significant key role in reversal learning. Reversal learning is the ability to alter behaviour when reinforcement contingencies change. Like the DLPFC and ACG, the VLPFC receives dopamine projections from the midbrain VTA via the mesocortical pathway. Substance-induced alterations in dopamine midbrain VTA signalling, therefore, will be communicated to the VLPFC (and the DLPFC and ACG). Such alterations are likely to have a detrimental impact on the integrity of cognitive control processes in these regions.

Substance addiction is characterized by continued use and recurrent relapse (despite serious negative consequences). Decrements, particularly in cognitive inhibitory control, may be a core feature of the disease and for which psychological and pharmacological treatments may be used to protect against relapse.

4.5 Putting it all together in addiction

Substances of abuse are rewarding. They are rewarding because they induce exaggerated increases in dopamine at the NAcc/VS. These increases alter the conscious experience of pleasure. These surges in dopamine-induced pleasure lead to 'liking'. The 'liking' of these substance-induced alterations in consciousness becomes powerfully connected to stimuli (i.e. cues) associated with the substance. These stimuli are robustly conditioned as abnormal memory traces connected to the pleasure and 'liking' of substance use. This conditioning involves a transition from 'liking' to 'wanting' the substance as addiction evolves.

Figure 4.2 Brain circuitry of addiction. Model of addiction as a result of chronic substance use within independent and overlapping circuits of the brain. Compared with the non-addicted circuitry (left), the salience value of a drug (red) and its associated cues (orange) becomes exaggerated in the addicted circuitry (right). The strength of inhibitory control is weakened (blue), together with unrestrained motivation/drive (green). This results in compulsive substance use and recurrent relapse in addiction.

Reprinted from *Trends in Molecular Medicine*, 12, Baler, R. D. & Volkow, N. D., Drug addiction: the neurobiology of disrupted self-control, pp. 559–566, Copyright (2006), with permission from Elsevier.

As the degree to which substance 'wanting' increases, the strength of inhibitory (No-go) control over reflexive, substance-taking behaviour is diminished (Go) as addiction develops (see Figure 4.2).

4.6 Conclusion

Anomalies within these circuits may also pre-date the addiction state and facilitate the progress from experimentation to substance addiction. The subsequent excessive and chronic use of substances further exacerbates these abnormalities. Therefore, reward, motivation and/or drive, learning and memory, and cognitive control are key processes to be understood if we are to develop and test new pharmacological and psychological treatment approaches in substance addiction.

FURTHER READING

Baler RD and Volkow ND (2006). Drug addiction: the neurobiology of disrupted self-control. *Trends in Molecular Medicine*, **12**, 559–66.

Crews FT and Boettiger CA (2009). Impulsivity, frontal lobes and risk for addiction. *Pharmacology Biochemistry and Behavior*, **93**, 237–47.

Goldstein RZ and Volkow ND (2011). Dysfunction of the prefrontal cortex in addiction: neuroimaging findings and clinical implications. *Nature Reviews Neuroscience*, **12**, 652–69.

Hyman SE (2005). Addiction: a disease of learning and memory. *American Journal of Psychiatry*, **162**, 1414–22.

Koob GF and Volkow ND (2010). Neurocircuitry of addiction. *Neuropsychopharmacology*, **35**, 217–38.

Verdejo-Garcia A and Bechara A (2009). A somatic marker theory of addiction. *Neuropharmacology*, **56 Suppl 1**, 48–62.

Volkow N and Fowler J (2000). Addiction, a disease of compulsion and drive: involvement of the orbitofrontal cortex. *Cerebral Cortex*, **10**, 318–25.

Volkow ND, Wang GJ, Fowler JS, et al. (2010). Addiction: decreased reward sensitivity and increased expectation sensitivity conspire to overwhelm the brain's control circuit. *Bioessays*, **32**, 748–55.

Volkow ND, Wang GJ, Fowler JS, et al. (2011). Addiction: beyond dopamine reward circuitry. *Proceedings of the National Academy of Sciences of the United States of America*, **108**, 15037–42.

CHAPTER 4

Drug pharmacokinetics and abuse liability

KEY POINTS

- Pharmacokinetics refers to the effect of the body on drugs.
- Pharmacokinetics predict the abuse liability of drugs.
- Route of administration (e.g. iv) predicts the speed at which drugs peak in plasma.
- Drugs that are quickly released have a greater abuse liability.
- The half-life of a drug can predict its reinforcing effects.
- Metabolism by the liver can predict a drug's reinforcing effects during withdrawal.

Pharmacokinetics refers to the effect of the body on drugs. Pharmacokinetics is divided into several areas, including the extent and rate of absorption, distribution, metabolism, and excretion of substances. Pharmacokinetics plays an important role in substance abuse. The speed at which different substances enter, act upon, and leave the brain plays a major role in the reinforcing effects, and abuse liability, of a substance.

5.1 Route of administration

The reinforcing effects of substances of addiction can be predicted by their route of administration (see Figure 5.1). Orally absorbed substances first pass into the stomach and then through the liver (the hepatic venous supply). The liver acts on the substance before it reaches other sites (e.g. brain). The liver will metabolize a significant proportion of the substance before it enters the systemic circulation—the 'first-pass' effect. This reduces the amount of the substance and delays its entry to the brain when taken orally.

Substances which are administered intravenously (iv) (e.g. cocaine, amphetamine, heroin) or smoked (e.g. crack cocaine, crystal methamphetamine, heroin), however, will reach the brain almost immediately—avoiding the 'first-pass' effect.

This rapid entry of a drug will mean there is more available and it will have an immediate pharmacological (e.g. increased dopamine) and subjective (e.g. pleasure) effect. This immediate and increased pleasurable effect is more reinforcing. For example, the rate (and dose) of iv cocaine has been shown to have a significant

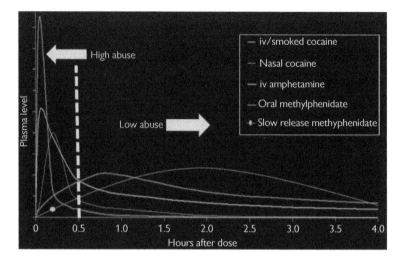

Figure 5.1 **Speed of brain entry predicts stimulant abuse.** The route of drug entry into the brain and its addiction potential. Drugs that are administered intravenously (iv) or smoked will enter the brain immediately to produce their reinforcing effects. This speed of entry confers a greater abuse liability.

influence on the intensity of reported positive subjective effects in experienced cocaine users. Indeed, iv (or smoked) cocaine are the two fastest routes for drug entry into the brain. These routes are associated with more self-reports for a greater loss of control over drug use, greater difficulty in reducing or stopping drug use, and an increased likelihood of developing addiction to the drug.

5.2 Drug onset

The abuse potential of amphetamines is related to their capacity to produce a rapid onset of presynaptic dopamine transporter (DAT) blockade in the brain. The pharmacokinetic effect of amphetamine (e.g. methylphenidate) has also been demonstrated in the brain. Immediate-release methylphenidate more rapidly occupies dopamine transporters. This more immediate occupancy of the dopamine transporter will expedite an increase in synaptic dopamine levels and ensuing subjective effects.

Therefore, the latency of methylphenidate's effects at the DAT and consequential dopamine increase are likely to influence the onset of positive subjective effects produced. This appears to be supported by the intensity of methylphenidate's onset of subjective effects. Immediate-release methylphenidate produces significantly higher subjective effects (e.g. positive, stimulant) compared to slow-release.

Therefore, the speed at which a drug can enter the brain and exert its pharmaco-logical effects is likely to confer greater abuse potential for that drug.

The reinforcing effects of substances can be predicted by how quickly the pleasurable effects of the substance are experienced. These effects may have a more rapid onset for some substances of abuse compared with others, irre-spective of method of administration (e.g. iv). This has been demonstrated in cocaine and methamphetamine addicts (see Figure 5.2). Cocaine, compared to methamphetamine, addicts report a more rapid onset of the subjective effects (e.g. 'high') following iv administration. The results also demonstrate how quickly the subjective effects for cocaine dissipate compared with that of methampheta-mine. This immediate onset, but short duration, of the subjective effects of co-caine likely contributes to its rapid reinforcing effects.

Figure 5.2 **The onset of subjective effects in cocaine and methamphetamine de-pendence.** Mean ratings for the onset and duration of self-reported 'high' for co-caine versus methamphetamine. Data are expressed as means and standard error. Significance is denoted by * (p <0.05), as indicated in the table below each panel.

Reprinted from *Pharmacology Biochemistry and Behavior*, 82, Newton, T. F., De La Garza, R., 2nd, Kalechstein, A. D., & Nestor, L. Cocaine and methamphetamine produce different patterns of subjective and cardiovascular effects, pp. 90–97. Copyright (2005), with permission from Elsevier.

There is also a close correlation between the rate at which substances of abuse enter and leave the brain and their reinforcing effects. For example, brain uptake for cocaine and its clearance in the ventral striatum (VS) are both very rapid (see Figures 5.3B and 5.3D). For methamphetamine, however, brain uptake and its clearance are both very slow in the VS compared to cocaine (see Figures 5.3A and 5.3C). Note the fast brain uptake for these drugs corresponds to the temporal course of the 'high'. This suggests that the 'high' is associated with a more rapid rate of dopamine increase at the VS. These different pharmacokinetic profiles

Figure 5.3 Pharmacokinetics parallel subjective effects of cocaine and methamphetamine. Pharmacokinetics of stimulant drugs in the human brain and relationship to self-reported 'high.' Axial brain images of the distribution of (A) [^{11}C]d-methamphetamine and (B) [^{11}C]cocaine at different times (minutes) after their administration. (C) Time activity curve for the concentration of [^{11}C]d-methamphetamine and (D) [^{11}C]cocaine alongside their respective temporal courses for the reported 'high' experienced after iv administration of these drugs.

Reprinted from *NeuroImage*, 43, Fowler, J. S., Volkow, N. D., Logan, J., et al. Fast uptake and long-lasting binding of methamphetamine in the human brain: comparison with cocaine. pp. 756–763, Copyright (2008), with permission from Elsevier.

may confer a quicker abuse liability for cocaine (particularly crack cocaine) but a greater neurotoxic effect profile for methamphetamine.

Functional MRI (fMRI) research has provided additional support regarding the onset and duration of cocaine in the brain. Brain regions (e.g. VTA, caudate, cingulate) that exhibit early and short duration levels of activity show a higher correlation with 'rush' ratings. In contrast, regions that demonstrate early but sustained activity are more correlated with craving (e.g. NAcc). These findings suggest that regions where iv cocaine induces rapid activation changes for short periods of time may act as the initial neural substrates of cocaine abuse.

5.3 Half-life

The half-life of a substance may additionally confer a greater abuse potential. Half-life is a measure of longevity in the tissue (e.g. plasma, brain) of a substance. It is defined as the time taken for its concentration to fall by one-half of the original concentration. The duration of action of methamphetamine (half-life ~11 hours), as opposed to cocaine (half-life ~90 minutes), for example, most likely influences patterns of self-administration in addicts—dosing is spaced throughout the day (methamphetamine) or is one of bingeing (cocaine). These patterns of use may be due to their durations of action, which are influenced by their half-lives.

5.4 Metabolism

Paradoxically, compounds that are more rapidly metabolized appear to be more difficult to stop using than those metabolized more slowly by the liver. For example, nicotine is metabolized extensively by the liver enzyme CYP2A6, primarily to cotinine. Cotinine is then metabolized by CYP2A6 to 3′-hydroxycotinine (3-HC). The higher ratio of metabolite to parent (i.e. 3-HC:cotinine), therefore, reflects greater CYP2A6 activity. Research has shown that smokers with higher CYP2A6 activity report greater ratings of nicotine-induced good **drug effects**, **drug liking**, and **drug wanting**. High metabolizers also report greater craving for cigarettes following overnight abstinence. These results suggest that the rate at which drugs of addiction are metabolized by the liver in some people, by accelerating withdrawal, may also confer a greater potential for abuse and dependence in those individuals.

5.5 Conclusion

Many substances of addiction work by triggering exaggerated increases in extracellular dopamine in the NAcc/VS. These increases resemble, and can greatly surpass, the physiological increases in dopamine triggered by naturally pleasurable stimuli. A rapid increase in the onset of a substance's pleasurable effects will make the substance more rewarding. This onset can be controlled by the route of substance administration (e.g. iv, smoked) and the speed the substance enters and leaves the brain (i.e. its clearance).

Evidence also suggests that rapid drug delivery is more effective in producing forms of neurobehavioural plasticity that may promote the transition from experimentation to addiction. The rapid delivery of drugs, like cocaine and nicotine, enhances their neurobiological effects in mesocorticolimbic structures (e.g. NAcc, OFC). This is thought to be an initial, and addiction-promoting, step leading to forms of drug-induced plasticity important for the evolution of addiction. The rate at which the body can metabolize a substance may also make it more reinforcing.

FURTHER READING

Breiter HC, Gollub RL, Weisskoff RM, et al. (1997). Acute effects of cocaine on human brain activity and emotion. *Neuron*, **19**, 591–611.

Fowler JS, Volkow ND, Logan J, et al. (2008). Fast uptake and long-lasting binding of methamphetamine in the human brain: comparison with cocaine. *Neuroimage*, **43**, 756–63.

Nelson RA, Boyd SJ, Ziegelstein RC, et al. (2006). Effect of rate of administration on subjective and physiological effects of intravenous cocaine in humans. *Drug and Alcohol Dependence*, **82**, 19–24.

Newton TF, De La Garza R 2nd, Kalechstein AD, et al. (2005). Cocaine and methamphetamine produce different patterns of subjective and cardiovascular effects. *Pharmacology Biochemistry and Behavior*, **82**, 90–7.

Parasrampuria DA, Schoedel KA, Schuller R, et al. (2007). Assessment of pharmacokinetics and pharmacodynamic effects related to abuse potential of a unique oral osmotic-controlled extended-release methylphenidate formulation in humans. *Journal of Clinical Pharmacology*, **47**, 1476–88.

Samaha AN, Li Y, and Robinson TE (2002). The rate of intravenous cocaine administration determines susceptibility to sensitization. *Journal of Neuroscience*, **22**, 3244–50.

Samaha AN and Robinson TE (2005). Why does the rapid delivery of drugs to the brain promote addiction? *Trends in Pharmacological Sciences*, **26**, 82–7.

Sofuoglu M, Herman AI, Nadim H et al. (2012). Rapid nicotine clearance is associated with greater reward and heart rate increases from intravenous nicotine. *Neuropsychopharmacology*, **37**, 1509–16.

Spencer TJ, Biederman J, Ciccone PE, et al. (2006). PET study examining pharmacokinetics, detection and likeability, and dopamine transporter receptor occupancy of short- and long-acting oral methylphenidate. *American Journal of Psychiatry*, **163**, 387–95.

CHAPTER 5

Pharmacodynamics of addictive substances

In Chapter 5, we were introduced to pharmacokinetics—the effect of the **body** on addictive substances. In this chapter, we will discuss pharmacodynamics—the effects of addictive substances on the body (i.e. in the brain). Acutely, addictive substances target various neurotransmitter systems in the brain (see Table 6.1). The pharmacological actions of these substances at receptors results in their physiological and behaviourally reinforcing effects.

The chronic use of addictive substances, however, leads to pharmacodynamic tolerance at receptors within neurotransmitter systems. This tolerance means that a greater amount of the substance is required to achieve the desired effect. This tolerance has significant implications for relapse during early abstinence which has led to new treatments that target various neurotransmitter systems which are disturbed in substance addiction.

6.1 Receptors

The acute and chronic effects of addictive substances essentially take place at receptors located within different neural networks of the brain. Receptors are proteins located on the cell membrane of neurons. Dopamine, for example, is a monoamine neurotransmitter which, when released from presynaptic neurons, binds with postsynaptic dopamine receptors to produce its physiological and behavioural effects.

The activation of some receptors by a neurotransmitter is coupled to biochemical transduction mechanisms in the postsynaptic neuron (i.e. second messengers). These are called G-protein coupled receptors, and adaptations at these receptors are complicit in substance addiction. Second messengers are chemicals

Table 6.1 Primary target and main effects of addictive substances in the brain

Drug	Primary target	Main effects	Other actions	Antagonists
Opiates	Stimulate mOR receptor	?	Stimulate delta and kappa opioid receptors	Naltrexone
Heroin				
Morphine/ methadone				
Buprenorphine	Less stimulation of mOR			
Stimulants				
Amphetamines	Promote dopamine release	Increase dopamine	Increase norepinephrine, serotonin, and endorphins	?
Cocaine	Blocks DAT	Increases dopamine	Inhibits norepinephrine reuptake	?
Nicotine	Stimulates nicotinic receptor	Increases dopamine		Mecamylamine
Sedatives				
Alcohol	Stimulate $GABA_A$ receptor	Increases GABA	Increases dopamine	?
		Reduces glutamate		
Benzodiazepines	Stimulate $GABA_A$ receptor	Increase GABA	?	Flumazenil
Gamma-hydroxybutyric acid	Stimulate $GABA_B$ and GHB receptors	Increases GABA	Increase dopamine	?

continued >

Cannabinoids				
Cannabis/marijuana	Stimulate CB$_1$ receptor	Increases dopamine	Reduces GABA and norepinephrine release	Rimonabant
Hallucinogenics				
Lysergic acid diethylamide	Stimulate serotinin 5-HT$_2$ receptor	Mimics serotonin	Increases dopamine	Ketanserin
				Ritanserin
MDMA	Promotes serotonin release	Increases serotonin	Increases dopamine	SSRIs (e.g. fluoxetine)
			Increases norepinephrine and serotonin?	

whose concentration increases or decreases in response to receptor activation by a neurotransmitter or drug. In the case of dopamine, binding to the D1/5R activates an enzyme called adenylyl cyclase. The activation of this enzyme increases the formation of a coenzyme called adenosine triphosphate (ATP). ATP catalyzes cyclic adenosine monophosphate (cAMP), leading to the activation of calcium (Ca^{2+}) channels.

Dopamine or agonist drugs binding to the D2/3/4R, however, have the opposite effect. This results in reduced formation of cAMP, as these receptors are negatively coupled to adenylyl cyclase. G-protein coupled receptors exert their effects slowly over seconds or minutes. Stimulants (e.g. cocaine, amphetamine), which are highly addictive in humans, are particularly powerful indirect agonists at these receptors as they increase synaptic dopamine. Addictive substances, such as cannabis and heroin/morphine, also exert their effects at G-protein coupled receptors in the brain.

Ligand-gated receptors (ionotropic or channel-linked receptors), on the other hand, are made up of protein subunits that form a central ion channel. The ion channel is regulated by a ligand (drug or neurotransmitter) and is usually very selective for one or more ions (e.g. Na$^+$, K$^+$, Ca^{2+}, or Cl$^-$). The stimulation of such receptors is converted into a postsynaptic electrical signal very rapidly (i.e. in the order of milliseconds). Nicotine, which is the main constituent of tobacco and highly addictive, exerts its acute effects within the brain by acting at ligand-gated nicotinic acetylcholine receptors (nAChRs). The nAChR is a Na^+ and K^+ ion channel. Likewise, alcohol, which is powerfully addictive, exerts its effects in the brain at fast-acting ligand-gated $GABA_A$ receptors. $GABA_A$ receptors conduct Cl^- ions.

6.2 Receptor agonists

Most addictive substances exert their effects directly (i.e. by mimicking a neurotransmitter) or indirectly (i.e. by modulating neurotransmitter activity) at specific receptors in the brain. The binding of an agonist to the receptor on the cell membrane of a neuron triggers a response in that neuron. Substances of addiction that act as direct agonists are alcohol, cannabis, heroin/morphine, and nicotine. When these substances are consumed and reach the brain, they interact directly with their receptors to elicit their intrinsic effects in the nerve cell.

Cocaine and amphetamine, however, act as indirect agonists at receptors. Following their consumption and entrance into the brain, they act to first increase the synaptic availability of the neurotransmitter (i.e. dopamine—and also norepinephrine and serotonin). Cocaine blocks the reuptake of synaptic dopamine by inhibiting the presynaptic dopamine transporter (DAT). Blocking the DAT inhibits the reuptake of dopamine in the presynaptic nerve terminal. Amphetamines (e.g. crystal methamphetamine) enter presynaptic nerve terminals and increase neurotransmitter release. The increased availability of these neurotransmitters by cocaine and amphetamines, therefore, induces a greater chemical/receptor interaction and, thus, a greater response in the nerve cell.

Certain agonists have been specifically developed to act as a substitute in the management and treatment of addiction. Methadone, for example, is an opioid receptor agonist used to manage heroin addiction. Methadone acts as a substitute for heroin as it is a full opioid agonist that mimics the actions of heroin (see Figure 6.1). Methadone, however, has a slower onset of effect and, when taken orally, is less reinforcing.

More recently, **partial agonist** replacement therapies for addiction (e.g. heroin) have been tested with a view to only partially stimulating receptors to reduce the risk of overdose. A partial agonist is a compound that activates the given receptor but has only partial efficacy at the receptor relative to a full agonist. Furthermore, the partial agonist also acts as a competitive antagonist in the presence of a full agonist. Here, it competes with the full agonist for receptor occupancy and produces a net decrease in receptor activation compared to that observed with the full agonist alone. For example, the partial mu opioid receptor agonist buprenorphine affords itself this mechanism of action (see Figure 6.1) and has become an alternative to methadone in the treatment and management of heroin addiction. Should a heroin-addicted individual decide to take methadone (or heroin) in the presence of buprenorphine, its effects would be blocked.

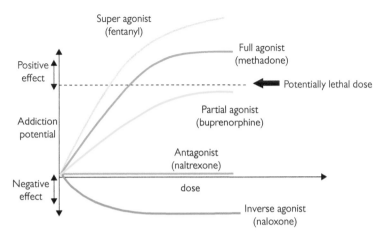

Figure 6.1 **Receptor activation.** Strength of receptor activation by a super, full, partial, and inverse agonist as well as an antagonist at the mu opioid receptor.

6.3 Efficacy

Intrinsic efficacy refers to the ability of an agonist to alter the conformation of a receptor. This efficacy is measured by the strength of the response elicited by the agonist. Also, the strength of this response acts as a predictor of efficacy for compounds (see Figure 6.1). Importantly, the more efficacious the agonist, the more potentially lethal it is when an overdose is taken.

6.4 Receptor antagonist

Antagonists are substances that have no intrinsic activity at receptors. They merely block an endogenous (i.e. neurotransmitter) or exogenous (i.e. drug) agonist from stimulating the receptor. While most addictive substances are agonists, there are substances that exert their effects (indirectly) by antagonizing (or blocking) certain receptors in the brain. Probably the best known of these substances are those that block the N-methyl D-aspartate (NMDA) receptor. NMDA receptor antagonists include (but are not limited to) ketamine (K), dextromethorphan (DXM), phencyclidine (PCP), and nitrous oxide (N_2O). These substances are popular recreational drugs due to their dissociative and hallucinogenic properties as well as their ability to induce euphoria.

Within the context of substance abuse and addiction, antagonists at different receptors in the brain have also been used to treat addiction. The mu opioid receptor antagonist naltrexone (see Figure 6.1), for example, is used for rapid detoxification (i.e. 'rapid detox') regimens for opioid dependence. Naltrexone has also been used to prevent relapse during the early stages of abstinence, given the emerging research evidence that the endorphin system is upregulated in substance addiction. Antagonists can also be added to agonists (e.g. buprenorphine + naltrexone) to reduce the risk of iv abuse.

6.5 Inverse agonists

Inverse agonists are compounds that bind to the same receptor as an agonist but instead induce a pharmacological response that is opposite to the agonist—they have negative efficacy. For example, the binding of an inverse agonist to a G-protein coupled receptor will induce the opposite response to that of an agonist in postsynaptic second messenger systems. The most common inverse agonist used in substance addiction is naloxone. Naloxone is used to counter the effects of opiate (e.g. heroin or morphine) overdose—specifically to counteract life-threatening depression within the respiratory centre of the brain (i.e. medulla oblongata).

6.6 Conclusion

Pharmacodynamics is the effect of substances or endogenous neurotransmitters at their receptors. Chronic substance use alters the functioning of neurotransmitter systems and their receptors—they can alter the pharmacodynamics of the brain. These changes in brain pharmacodynamics have significant implications for the effects of medications which are used to manage and treat substance addiction. Genetic polymorphisms at receptors in the brain, however, may alter pharmacodynamics and predispose some individuals to addiction.

FURTHER READING

Boileau I, Assaad JM, Pihl RO, et al. (2003). Alcohol promotes dopamine release in the human nucleus accumbens. *Synapse*, **49**, 226–31.

Bossong MG, van Berckel BN, Boellaard R, et al. (2009). Delta 9-tetrahydrocannabinol induces dopamine release in the human striatum. *Neuropsychopharmacology*, **34**, 759–66.

Nutt DJ (2010). Antagonist-agonist combinations as therapies for heroin addiction: back to the future? *Journal of Psychopharmacology*, **24(2)**, 141–5.

Rosa-Neto P, Gjedde A, Olsen AK, et al. (2004). MDMA-evoked changes in [11C] raclopride and [11C]NMSP binding in living pig brain. *Synapse*, **53**, 222–33.

Schiffer WK, Volkow ND, Fowler JS, et al. (2006). Therapeutic doses of amphetamine or methylphenidate differentially increase synaptic and extracellular dopamine. *Synapse*, **59**, 243–51.

Sirohi S, Dighe SV, Madia PA et al. (2009). The relative potency of inverse opioid agonists and a neutral opioid antagonist in precipitated withdrawal and antagonism of analgesia and toxicity. *Journal of Pharmacology and Experimental Therapeutics*, **330**, 513–19.

CHAPTER 7

The dopamine system and addiction

KEY POINTS

- Dopamine release is involved in the reinforcing effects of addictive substances.
- Dopamine release can be blunted by substance abuse.
- Dopamine release is involved in drug craving.
- Dopamine receptors are reduced during substance addiction withdrawal.
- Medications that boost dopamine functioning may be useful in substance addiction.
- Reductions in dopamine functioning may predispose people to substance addiction.

It has long been held that the reinforcing effects of substances of abuse involve the release of dopamine from presynaptic neurons of the ventral tegmental are (VTA) onto dopamine receptors (D1/2/3R) in the ventral striatum (VS). There is evidence, however, that not all drugs of abuse (e.g. opiates) increase the release of dopamine in humans. Research using animal models also suggests that dopamine functioning in the brain may predispose some individuals to initiating substance use—particularly the use of stimulants, which induce further deficits within the dopamine system.

In this chapter, we will examine the acute and chronic effects of addictive substances on the dopamine system. The potential efficacy of treatments that specifically target dopamine functioning in substance abuse and addiction will also be discussed.

7.1 The dopamine system

Dopamine is transmitted via three major pathways in the brain (see Figure 7.1). The first pathway extends from the substantia nigra (SN) to the caudate nucleus-putamen (neostriatum) and is concerned with sensory stimuli and movement. The second pathway projects from the ventral tegmental area (VTA) to the mesolimbic forebrain and is thought to be associated with cognitive, reward, and emotional behaviour. The third pathway, known as the tubero-infundibular system, is concerned with neuronal control of the hypothalmic-pituitary endocrine system.

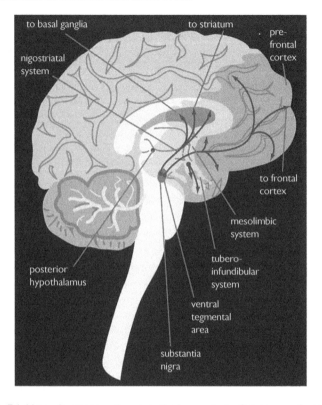

Figure 7.1 Major dopamine pathways in the human brain. Substances of addiction have a particularly strong influence on the pathway projecting from the ventral tegmental area (VTA) to the mesolimbic system containing the nucleus accumbens (NAcc)/ventral striatum (VS).

Substances of addiction work by triggering transient, exaggerated increases in dopamine at the VS. These surges in dopamine resemble, and can greatly surpass, physiological increases triggered by natural rewards (e.g. food, water). The two main substances of abuse that trigger exaggerated increases in dopamine are cocaine and amphetamines.

Cocaine is a reuptake inhibitor that binds to the presynaptic dopamine transporter (DAT). The DAT is a membrane-spanning protein located in subcortical regions of the brain, particularly in the striatum. It is responsible for sequestering extracellular dopamine back into presynaptic nerve terminals. By binding to the DAT on VTA neurons, for example, cocaine inhibits the reuptake of released dopamine at the VS (see Figure 7.2—cocaine). Amphetamines enter

Figure 7.2 Pharmacology of cocaine and amphetamines on dopamine. The effects of cocaine at the presynaptic DAT and amphetamine within the presynaptic neuron—both drug classes block reuptake, and amphetamines additionally stimulate dopamine release from nerve terminals. These increased levels of dopamine stimulate postsynaptic dopamine receptors, which produce the reinforcing effects of these substances (e.g. pleasure).

the presynaptic nerve terminal to promote the release of dopamine. This is done by interfering with vesicular storage and promoting carrier-mediated exchange. Amphetamines induce a surge in the release of dopamine from VTA neurons, leading to an increase in synaptic dopamine at the VS (see Figure 7.2—amphetamine). Amphetamines also inhibit the reuptake of dopamine to a lesser degree.

7.2 Substance addiction

The increase in dopamine by stimulants (and other substances) induces feelings of pleasure. One of the first studies to confirm these effects in humans showed that the resulting 'high' and 'rush' that people reported was directly related to dopamine at the D2R (see Figure 7.3).

Due to the surges in dopamine release by substances of abuse, chronic use may result in a pathological shift in the hedonic set point during addiction. This state of dysregulation within evolutionary hard-wired brain reward systems has been demonstrated using a number of different methods. For example, evidence suggests that there are significantly **fewer** D2/3R numbers in cocaine and alcohol dependence (see Figure 7.4).

In addition to D2R reductions in substance-dependent populations, there is also evidence for reduced dopamine release in addiction. Using an amphetamine

Figure 7.3 Dopamine release and the subjective effects of amphetamine. (A) [C-11] raclopride displacement from the D2R by methylphenidate-induced dopamine release in the VS. The colour scale (from red to blue) represents the amount of [C-11] raclopride emission decreasing, as it is displaced by increasing levels of dopamine related to the dose of methylphenidate. (B) Correlations between methylphenidate-induced changes in D2R availability in the VS as an effect of dose and methylphenidate-induced changes in self-reports of high ($r = 0.78$, df_{22}, $p < 0.0001$) and rush ($r = 0.75$, $p < 0.0001$).

Adapted from *Journal of Pharmacology and Experimental Therapeutics*, 291, 1, Volkow, N. D., Wang, G. J., Fowler, et al., Reinforcing effects of psychostimulants in humans are associated with increases in brain dopamine and occupancy of D(2) receptors, pp. 409–415. © 1999 American Society for Pharmacology & Experimental Therapeutics.

challenge (e.g. methylphenidate administration), it has been shown that cocaine abusers exhibit an attenuated dopamine response in the VS compared to controls (see Figure 7.5). This effect has also been reported in alcohol, heroin, and methamphetamine dependence. The deficit in dopamine release may confer an additional vulnerability to relapse and bingeing in an attempt to overcome this hedonic dysregulation.

Paradoxically, cocaine cues (e.g. objects, people, places associated with the rewarding effects of cocaine) significantly **increase** dopamine release in the **dorsal striatum** (DS) in cocaine dependence. The magnitude of this

Reduced dopamine D2/3 receptor levels have
been found in alcohol and cocaine dependence:

Overall reduction: 10% in Alcohol and 12% in Cocaine studies.

NB: For opioids, nicotine, cannabis - robust consistent
reductions in dopamine receptor levels have NOT been found.

Figure 7.4 **Reduced D2/3R numbers in substance addiction.** The graph shows the results (unpublished) from a meta-analysis of previously published research on D2/3R numbers in alcohol and cocaine addiction.

effect is also highly correlated with the subjective experience of craving (see Figure 7.6).

The DS has been implicated in habit learning, as substance abuse progresses. Research also suggests that behavioural changes in addiction are represented by a transition from cortical to subcortical (i.e. striatal) control and, within the striatum, from the VS to the DS (i.e. caudate). Therefore, conditioned cues trigger reflexive, exaggerated surges in dopamine release.

Research also suggests that reduced dopamine transmission, in addiction, might actually predict treatment failure. Patients with low methylphenidate-induced dopamine release respond less favourably to behavioural treatment that uses positive reinforcement to reduce impulsive cocaine use (Martinez et al. 2012).

These findings cannot rule out the possibility of dopamine deficits prior to substance abuse and dependence. Research in animals, for example, suggests a role for the D2R with respect to impulsivity and, consequently, the development of cocaine abuse. High impulsive rats have lower D2R levels in the VS and self-administer cocaine (but not heroin) significantly more than low impulsive rats. Social status in monkeys is also associated with D2R levels and cocaine abuse. Lower social status is associated with fewer D2R and greater cocaine self-administration. If the social status of an animal is reversed, so are D2R levels and cocaine intake.

Figure 7.5 Reduced dopamine release in substance addiction. Dopamine release induced by methylphenidate (MP) in controls and active cocaine-addicted subjects. (A) Average non-displaceable binding of [¹¹C] raclopride after placebo and after MP (iv). The colour scale (from red to blue) represents the amount of [¹¹C]raclopride emission decreasing, as it is displaced by increasing levels of dopamine related to MP. (B) D2R availability in the caudate, putamen, and VS after placebo (blue) and after MP (red) in controls and cocaine-addicted subjects. Note that cocaine abusers show both decreases in baseline striatal D2R availability (placebo measure) and decreases in dopamine release when given MP (measured as decreases in D2R availability from baseline).

Reproduced from *Proceedings of the National Academy of Sciences*, 108, 37, Volkow, N. D., Wang, G. J., Fowler, J. S., Tomasi, D., Telang, F., Addiction: beyond dopamine reward circuitry, pp. 15037–15042, 2011 National Academy of Sciences, USA.

7.3 Treatment

Research examining potential treatment approaches to substance addiction has involved the use of compounds that modulate dopamine functioning (see Table 7.1). This research has involved the assessment of abstinence and particularly the efficacy of these compounds to reduce the subjective effects and craving that are induced by small, priming doses of a substance (e.g. alcohol, amphetamine, cocaine).

The partial D2R agonist **aripiprazole** may possess some efficacy in reducing alcohol intake and increasing abstinence from alcohol (Voronin et al. 2008). Aripiprazole blocks the effects of dopamine when they are high but augments dopamine when it is low. This may, therefore, be beneficial in both reducing dopamine tone (e.g. during craving in response to cues) and increasing dopamine tone (e.g. during low mood and anhedonia). Aripiprazole also attenuates activation in the VS of alcoholics in response to alcohol cues and reduces the reinforcing

Figure 7.6 **Craving-induced dopamine release in substance addiction**. Dopamine changes induced by conditioned cues in active cocaine abusers. (A) Average non-displaceable binding potential of [¹¹C]raclopride in cocaine-addicted subjects tested while viewing a neutral video (nature scenes) and while viewing a cocaine video (i.e. people administering cocaine). The colour scale (from red to blue) represents the amount of [¹¹C] raclopride emission decreasing in areas where there is more dopamine binding to the D2R. (B) D2R availability in the DS (i.e. caudate), pu-tamen, and VS for the neutral video (blue) and the cocaine cues video (red). Cocaine cues significantly increased dopamine in the caudate and putamen but not in the VS. (C) Correlation between changes in D2R and cocaine craving induced by the cocaine video.

Reproduced from *Proceedings of the National Academy of Sciences of the United States of America*, 108, 37, Volkow, N. D., Wang, G. J., Fowler, J. S. et al, Addiction: beyond dopamine reward circuitry, pp. 15037–15042.Copyright (2011) the Authors. Published by National Academy of Sciences, USA. Source data from *Journal of Neuroscience*, 26, Volkow, N.D, Wang G.J., Cocaine cues and dopamine in dorsal striatum: Mechanism of craving in cocaine addiction, 2006.

subjective effects (e.g. **good effect, like, willing to take again**) of amphet-amine in stimulant abusers (Lile et al. 2005).

Bupropion inhibits the reuptake of dopamine and enhances residual dopa-mine neurotransmission. Research has shown that it attenuates the reinforcing effects of methamphetamine and reduces methamphetamine craving (Newton et al. 2006). This effect appears to be due to bupropion's inhibition of metham-phetamine uptake—limiting the ability of methamphetamine to displace vesicular dopamine. The inhibition of dopamine uptake at the DAT may ameliorate the methamphetamine abstinence syndrome. Bupropion has not demonstrated any efficacy for cocaine dependence, however.

Table 7.1 Dopamine-modulating compounds that have been tested as potential treatments for substance addiction

Medication	Mechanism of action	Addiction type	Efficacy
Amantadine	Dopamine releaser	Cocaine	Not effective and its discontinuation may increase in cocaine use
			Does not reduce preference for cocaine
			May reduce the desire to use cocaine when combined with the GABA$_B$ agonist baclofen
			May be effective in patients with severe cocaine withdrawal symptoms
Aripiprazole	Partial D2R agonist	Alcohol	May reduce drinking in those with lower self-control
			Less efficacious than naltrexone for craving
			Attenuates ventral striatal activation in response to alcohol cues
		Amphetamine	Reduces subjective effects of amphetamine challenge
		Cocaine	Increases cocaine self-administration
		Methamphetamine	Increases rewarding effects of acute methamphetamine
Bupropion	DAT inhibitor	Cocaine	Does not alter the acute subjective effects of cocaine
			May enhance the positive subjective effects of cocaine
		Methamphetamine	Reduces the positive subjective effects of methamphetamine
			Reduces cue-induced craving

continued >

Disulfiram	Dopamine β-hydroxylase inhibitor	Alcohol	Deters alcohol consumption
		Cocaine	Reduces the positive subjective effects of cocaine
			Weight-based medication doses negatively predict the preference for cocaine
Levodopa	Dopamine precursor	Cocaine	No effect on cocaine use, craving, or mood
Methamphetamine	Dopamine releaser	Cocaine	Methamphetamine SR reduces cocaine use and craving
Methylphenidate	Dopamine releaser	Cocaine	Enhances anterior cingulate activation and reduces impulsive responding
			Oral slow release decreases the reinforcing effects of cocaine in those with ADHD
			Provides no advantage over placebo in reducing cocaine use
		Methamphetamine	No different to placebo in reducing methamphetamine use
Modafinil	DAT inhibitor	Alcohol	May improve state impulsivity in those with poor response inhibition
		Cocaine	In combination with individual behavioural therapy may reduce cocaine use
		Methamphetamine	Does not reduce methamphetamine use
			May reduce the acute reinforcing effects of methamphetamine

continued >

Table 7.1 Dopamine-modulating compounds that have been tested as potential treatments for substance addiction *(continued)*

Selegiline	Monoamine oxidase B Inhibitor	Cocaine	No significant effect over placebo in reducing cocaine use
		Methamphetamine	May increase negative subjective effects of acute methamphetamine

Disulfiram inhibits aldehyde dehydrogenase, resulting in acetaldehyde accumulation. This produces symptoms of hypotension, diaphoresis, flushing, nausea, and vomiting in response to alcohol consumption during drinking. This reaction is aimed at making alcohol use negatively reinforcing. There are currently no medications approved for the treatment of cocaine dependence. Disulfiram is also a dopamine β-hydroxylase inhibitor—it prevents the conversion of dopamine to norepinephrine in presynaptic nerve terminals, thus increasing vesicular dopamine stores. Research suggests that disulfiram may possess some clinical efficacy during cocaine relapse, as it significantly attenuates the reinforcing effects (e.g. reported **high, rush**) of cocaine compared to placebo (Baker et al. 2007).

Substance addiction is associated with dysregulated dopaminergic transmission. This dysregulation of the dopamine system may also result in functional impairments in regions heavily innervated by dopamine, such as the prefrontal cortex (PFC). The PFC is essential to higher-order cognitive processing, such as impulse control. Therefore, medications that enhance dopamine functioning in the PFC may confer increased cognitive control over impulsive and risk-taking behaviours, such as substance use.

Methylphenidate has been shown to improve inhibitory control and decrease abnormal risk-taking in adolescents with attention deficit hyperactive disorder (ADHD). Compared to placebo, it has also been shown to significantly reduce impulsivity while, at the same time, enhance activation in the anterior cingulate gyrus (ACG) in cocaine abusers (Goldstein et al. 2010). Interestingly, this effect was found in the dorsal-cognitive division of the ACG, suggesting that methylphenidate may augment the neural cognitive control over impulsivity. While methylphenidate may be efficacious in those with ADHD and cocaine dependence, its efficacy in other non-ADHD populations with addictions remains to be fully tested.

7.4 Conclusion

Reward is a central component for driving incentive-based learnings. Substances of abuse are rewarding because they induce the release of dopamine in evolutionary hard-wired neural circuitry that is critical for survival-based behaviours. Chronic substance use, however, can induce a pathological shift in the responsiveness of this circuitry in response to both natural and substance reinforcers. Medications that augment dopamine functioning may be helpful in the treatment of substance addiction—particularly in reducing impulsivity and the acute reinforcing effects of substances upon relapse. There may be deficits in dopamine reward functioning, however, that predate substance abuse and addiction.

FURTHER READING

Baker JR, Jatlow P, and McCance-Katz EF (2007). Disulfiram effects on responses to intravenous cocaine administration. *Drug and Alcohol Dependence*, **87**, 202–9.

Dackis CA, Kampman KM, Lynch KG, et al.# (2005). A double-blind, placebo-controlled trial of modafinil for cocaine dependence. *Neuropsychopharmacology*, **30**, 205–11.

Goldstein RZ and Volkow ND (2002). Drug addiction and its underlying neurobiological basis: neuroimaging evidence for the involvement of the frontal cortex. *American Journal of Psychiatry*, **159**, 1642–52.

Goldstein RZ, Woicik PA, Maloney T, et al. (2010). Oral methylphenidate normalizes cingulate activity in cocaine addiction during a salient cognitive task. *Proceedings of the National Academy of Science of the United States of America*, **107**, 16667–72.

Heal DJ, Smith SL, Gosden J, et al. (2013). Amphetamine, past and present—a pharmacological and clinical perspective. *Journal of Psychopharmacology*, **27**(**6**), 479–96.

Lile JA, Stoops WW, Vansickel AR, et al. (2005). Aripiprazole attenuates the discriminative-stimulus and subject-rated effects of D-amphetamine in humans. *Neuropsychopharmacology*, **30**, 2103–14.

Martinez D, Carpenter KM, Liu F, et al. (2012). Imaging dopamine transmission in cocaine dependence: link between neurochemistry and response to treatment. *American Journal of Psychiatry*, **168**, 634–41.

Newton TF, Roache JD, De La Garza R, 2nd, et al. (2006). Bupropion reduces methamphetamine-induced subjective effects and cue-induced craving. *Neuropsychopharmacology*, **31**, 1537–44.

Volkow ND, Wang GJ, Fowler JS, et al. (1999). Reinforcing effects of psychostimulants in humans are associated with increases in brain dopamine and occupancy of D(2) receptors. *Journal of Pharmacology and Experimental Therapeutics*, **291**, 409–15.

Volkow ND, Wang GJ, Telang F, et al. (2007). Profound decreases in dopamine release in striatum in detoxified alcoholics: possible orbitofrontal involvement. *Journal of Neuroscience*, **27**, 12700–6.

Volkow ND, Wang GJ, Fowler JS, et al. (2011). Addiction: beyond dopamine reward circuitry. *Proceedings of the National Academy of Sciences of the United States of America*, **108**, 15037–42.

Voronin K, Randall P, Myrick H, et al. (2008). Aripiprazole effects on alcohol consumption and subjective reports in a clinical laboratory paradigm—possible influence of self-control. *Alcoholism: Clinical and Experimental Research*, **32**, 1954–61.

CHAPTER 8

The GABA system and addiction

KEY POINTS

- GABA is the major inhibitory neurotransmitter in the brain.
- GABA binds with $GABA_A$ and $GABA_B$ receptors to inhibit neuronal activity.
- Substances of abuse can downregulate or upregulate the GABA system.
- $GABA_B$ receptors modulate substance reward and reinforcement behaviours.
- Disturbances to the GABA system may pre-date substance addiction.
- Compounds that target the GABA system may help in the treatment of addiction.

Substances of addiction impinge upon, and disrupt, a variety of neurotransmitter systems in the brain. Research has recently pointed to the potential role of gamma-aminobutyric acid (GABA) in substance abuse and dependence (see Figure 8.1). GABA is the major inhibitory neurotransmitter in the brain. Deficits in the functioning of this system may alter its efficacy to modulate other neurotransmitter systems (e.g. dopamine), which are strongly implicated in substance addiction.

In this chapter, we will discuss the potential role of GABA in substance addiction and the potential value of compounds that target this system in the treatment and management of substance use disorders.

8.1 The GABA system

GABAergic inhibition is seen at all levels of the brain, including the hypothalamus, hippocampus, frontal cortex, nucleus accumbens (NAcc), and cerebellum. As well as the large well-established GABA pathways, GABA interneurons are abundant in the brain, with ~50% of all inhibitory synapses in the brain mediated by GABA.

GABA is synthesized from glutamate and, when released, binds with two types of receptors. The first are ionotropic $GABA_A$ receptors that contain chloride ion channels. These receptors predominately mediate rapid inhibitory neurotransmission throughout the brain via an influx of chloride ions (see Figure 8.2).

Chloride ion influx hyperpolarizes the neuron cell membrane—it induces neuronal inhibition. $GABA_A$ receptors consist of several glycoprotein subunits (or binding sites). Substances, such as benzodiazepines, barbiturates, steroids, alcohol, and general anaesthetics, have different affinities for these subunits. GABA also activates a class of metabotropic $GABA_B$ receptors (see Figure 8.2).

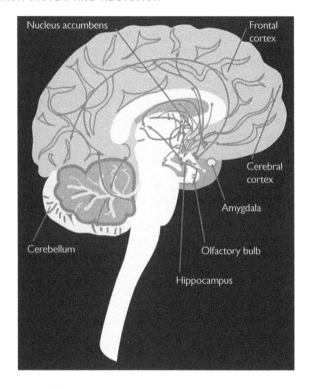

Figure 8.1 Major GABA pathways in the human brain. GABA exerts its inhibitory effect on other neurotransmitter systems, mainly through GABAergic interneurons.

GABA$_B$ receptors are located on both pre- and postsynaptic neurons: presynaptic receptors typically inhibit the release of other neurotransmitters whereas postsynaptic receptors are excitatory. GABA$_B$ receptors are thought to modulate a variety of substance use-related reward and reinforcement behaviours.

GABA exerts its inhibitory effect on other neurotransmitter systems, mainly through GABAergic interneurons. For example, interneurons in the ventral tegmental area (VTA) are a primary inhibitory regulator of dopamine neurons projecting to the ventral striatum (VS). Substances that inhibit these interneurons, such as heroin at the mu opioid receptor, therefore, reduce GABAergic inhibition of VTA dopamine neuron projections to the VS. Moreover, a subset of GABAergic medium spiny neurons in the VS send reciprocal projections back to the VTA—a projection that mediates inhibitory feedback on dopamine neuron activity via GABA$_B$ receptors.

Figure 8.2 The neurochemistry of GABA, showing (1) the synthesis of GABA from glutamate (via glutamic acid decarboxylase; (2) transport and storage of GABA in the vesicle; (3) the release of GABA by exocytosis; (4) binding to ionotropic GABA$_A$ receptors and the influx of chloride ions (Cl$^-$) that hyperpolarize the nerve cell; (5) binding to metabotropic GABA$_B$ receptors and subsequent downstream effects mediated via a G-protein and/or cAMP to K$^+$ and Na$^+$ channels; and (6) the reuptake of synaptic GABA into the presynaptic nerve terminal.

Medium spiny GABAergic neurons are also the principal projection neurons of the striatum. They receive excitatory glutamatergic inputs from the cerebral cortex and thalamus and modulatory dopaminergic innervation from the midbrain VTA. Striatopallidal medium spiny neurons express the dopamine 2 receptor (D2R) whereas striatonigral medium spiny neurons express the dopamine

1 receptor (D1R). These two sets of GABAergic neurons are homogenously distributed throughout the striatum and are known to have opposing behavioural effects—striatonigral is part of the 'direct pathway', and the striatopallidal is part of the 'indirect pathway'.

Therefore, the GABA systems within midbrain and striatal regions are well placed to accommodate the modulating effects of substances of addiction and the potential of medications to modify activity in these regions during treatment.

8.2 Substance addiction

There are a number of abused substances that boost GABA functioning. These are typically the sedative or 'downer' substances, such as alcohol, benzodiazepines, gammahydroxybutyrate (GHB), and barbiturates—all enhance the actions of GABA at the $GABA_A$ receptor to sedate the brain. Evidence suggests, however, that stimulants may also influence GABA functioning indirectly, perhaps sensitizing the GABA system following chronic use (Volkow et al. 1998).

The α5 subtype of the GABA-benzodiazepine receptor is thought to play a prominent and specific role in the reinforcing effects of alcohol. This is due to its distribution in striatal regions of the brain and the efficacy of agonists and antagonists to increase and decrease, respectively, alcohol self-administration in animals. The α5 subtype is significantly lower in the nucleus accumbens (NAc)/VS of abstinent alcoholics (see Figure 8.3) as well as in the hippocampus and amygdala. This finding may suggest the α5 subtype downregulates in limbic brain regions in order to compensate for the chronic effects of alcohol. Benzodiazepine receptor distribution is also significantly lower in frontal regions of the brain in alcoholics.

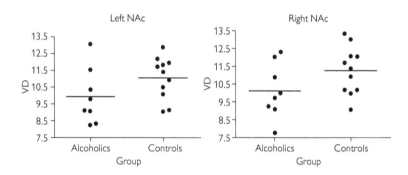

Figure 8.3 Reduced striatal GABA benzodiazepine receptors in alcoholics, showing the spread of the α5 GABA-benzodiazepine receptor subtype in the left and right nucleus accumbens (NAc) in abstinent alcoholic patients and controls.

Reproduced from *Journal of Psychopharmacology*, 26, 2, Lingford-Hughes, A., Reid, .A. G., Myers, J. et al., A [11C]Ro15 4513 PET study suggests that alcohol dependence in man is associated with reduced α5 benzodiazepine receptors in limbic regions, pp. 273–281. Copyright © 2012, © SAGE Publications

These results in alcoholism and cocaine addiction may point to the opposing long-term effects of these substances on GABA functioning.

8.3 Treatment

The benzodiazepines, such as diazepam, are the most commonly used compounds for managing alcohol withdrawal. Their long-term use, however, is not recommended, given their interaction with alcohol and their abuse potential. Research suggests that **baclofen** (30 mg/day), a selective GABA$_B$ receptor agonist, may be as effective as diazepam for alcohol withdrawal (see Figure 8.4).

There are also concerns regarding interactions between benzodiazepines and **opioid** medications (e.g. methadone and buprenorphine). Benzodiazepines and opiates interact to induce increased levels of subjective effects (i.e. abuse potential) and sedation (see Figure 8.5). Benzodiazepines are also frequently identified at autopsy in methadone-related deaths.

Research has also tested the potential efficacy of GABA compounds to reduce relapse and attenuate the acute reinforcing effects of substances—thereby suggesting a potential role for GABA in substance abuse and dependence treatment (see

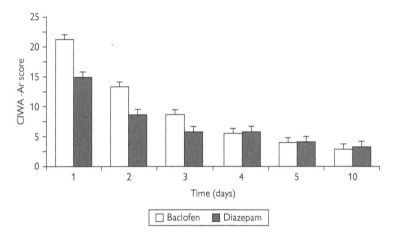

Figure 8.4 **Baclofen reduces alcohol withdrawal.** Score of the Clinical Institute Withdrawal Assessment for Alcohol-revised (CIWA-Ar) scale in patients treated for 10 consecutive days with baclofen (30 mg/day) and diazepam (0.5–0.75 mg/kg/day on days 1–6, tapering the dose by 25% daily from day 7 to day 10. CIWA-Ar administration occurred once a day, on days 1, 2, 3, 4, 5, and 10, immediately before the first daily administration of drugs (scoring of day 1 is baseline).

Figure 8.5 Pharmacodynamic interactions of diazepam with opiates. Visual analogue scale ratings (0–100 mm) of sedation (not sedated–very sedated) and liking of drug effect (dislike very much–like very much), following administration of either 0 mg diazepam (0 mg DIAZ) or 40 mg diazepam (40 mg DIAZ), in combination with either 100% or 150% of the normal maintenance opioid dose (100% OP/150% OP) of methadone or buprenorphine. Data are expressed as mean ± SEM.

Reprinted from *Drug and Alcohol Dependence*, 91, Lintzeris, N., Mitchell, T. B., Bond, A. J., et al. Pharmacodynamics of diazepam co-administered with methadone or buprenorphine under high dose conditions in opioid dependent patients, pp. 187–194, Copyright (2007), with permission from Elsevier.

Table 8.1). Baclofen, the GABA$_B$ agonist, has also proven potentially efficacious in preventing alcohol lapse and relapse in alcoholics with liver cirrhosis (see Figure 8.6).

Tiagabine is a GABA reuptake inhibitor—its mechanism of action makes more GABA available for synaptic transmission (see (6) in Figure 8.2). Tiagabine

Table 8.1 GABA-modulating compounds that have been tested as potential treatments for substance addiction. GAD, glutamate decarboxylase; GABA-T, GABA-transaminase.

Medication	Mechanism of action	Addiction type	Efficacy
Baclofen	GABA$_B$ agonist	Alcohol	Suppresses alcohol withdrawal syndrome
			Produces a decrease in alcohol craving when prescribed with no superior limit of dose
			Shows a dose–effect relationship in reducing alcohol use
			Associated with a significant reduction in state anxiety in alcoholics
			Well tolerated and safe when given in combination with intoxicating doses of alcohol
		Cocaine	Attenuates cocaine relapse in baboons
			May reduce some positive reinforcing effects of cocaine when combined with amantadine
			Reduces self-administration of cocaine
			Reduces craving in methadone-maintained patients also dependent on cocaine
		Methamphetamine	May have a small treatment effect relative to placebo
Tiagabine	GABA reuptake inhibitor	Alcohol	May be effective in alcohol dependence when combined with standard psychotherapy
		Cocaine	Does not attenuate cocaine relapse in baboons
			Attenuates craving and some of the reinforcing effects of acute cocaine administration

continued >

Table 8.1 GABA-modulating compounds that have been tested as potential treatments for substance addiction. GAD, glutamate decarboxylase; GABA-T, GABA-transaminase. *(continued)*

			Reduces cocaine-taking compared to placebo or gabapentin in methadone-maintained users
			Dose of 20 mg/day does not robustly decrease cocaine use
			Does not alter the effects of oral cocaine
Topiramate	GABA$_A$ agonist?	Alcohol	Reduces alcohol craving and increases alcohol abstinence
			Potential efficacy for relapse prevention
			May be superior to naltrexone in reducing alcohol craving
			May reduce subjective effects of alcohol more than alcohol craving
			Up to 300 mg/d superior to placebo in lessening dependence severity and harmful drinking
		Cocaine	May be effective in promoting cocaine abstinence
		Methamphetamine	Does not appear to promote abstinence but can reduce amount of methamphetamine used
			May enhance, rather than attenuate, the positive subjective effects of methamphetamine
Valproate	GAD inducer and inhibitor of GABA-T	Cocaine	Does not reduce spontaneous and cue-induced cocaine craving
Vigabatrin	Inhibitor of GABA-T	Cocaine	Short-term use may increase abstinence from cocaine
		Methamphetamine	Not efficacious in attenuating the positive subjective effects of methamphetamine in the laboratory

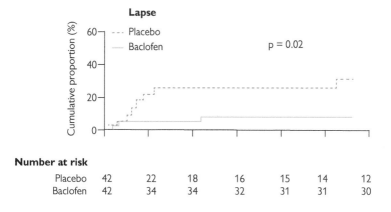

Number at risk

Placebo	42	22	18	16	15	14	12
Baclofen	42	34	34	32	31	31	30

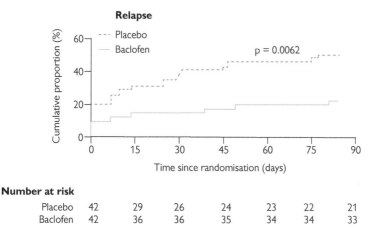

Number at risk

Placebo	42	29	26	24	23	22	21
Baclofen	42	36	36	35	34	34	33

Figure 8.6 **Baclofen reduces relapse risk in alcoholics.** Survival analysis of proportion of lapse and relapse in alcoholics. Number at risk refers to proportion remaining free of lapse and relapse. Cumulative abstinence duration was about twofold higher in patients allocated to baclofen than in those assigned to placebo (mean 62·8 ± 5·4] vs 30·8 ± 5.5 days; p = 0·001). No hepatic side effects were recorded.

Reprinted from *The Lancet*, 370, Addolorato, G., Leggio, L., Ferrulli, A. et al. Effectiveness and safety of baclofen for maintenance of alcohol abstinence in alcohol-dependent patients with liver cirrhosis: randomised, double-blind controlled study, pp. 1915–1922. Copyright (2007), with permission from Elsevier.

Figure 8.7 Tiagabine reduces the effects of cocaine. Tiagabine effects on average subjective responses, using the Cocaine Effects Questionnaire (CEQ), to iv saline and two escalating doses of cocaine (0.15 and 0.3 mg/kg), given 30 min apart. The measurements were obtained 4.5 min before and 2.5, 10, and 15 min after saline and cocaine administration. Data shown are the average values (SEM) and significant group difference (p <0.05) for craving and stimulated.

Reprinted from *Pharmacology Biochemistry and Behavior*, 82, Sofuoglu, M., Poling, J., Mitchell, E., & Kosten, T. R., Tiagabine affects the subjective responses to cocaine in humans, pp. 569–573. Copyright (2005), with permission from Elsevier.

has been reported to attenuate craving and some of the subjective effects of iv cocaine (see Figure 8.7). Results suggest that it does not attenuate the effects of oral cocaine, however.

Tiagabine may also be more clinically effective than placebo or gabapentin in reducing cocaine use in methadone-maintained cocaine abusers (see Figure 8.8). For alcohol dependence, tiagabine has shown some efficacy when combined with standard psychotherapy.

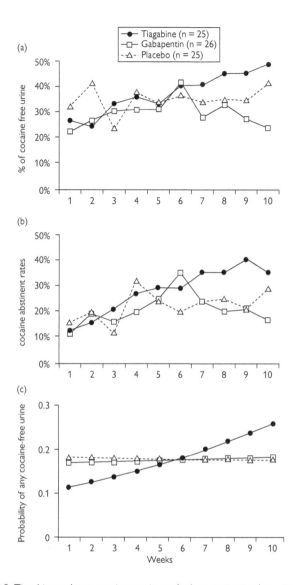

Figure 8.8 Tiagabine reduces cocaine use in methadone-maintained cocaine abusers. (a) Change of the percentage of cocaine-free urines per week by treatment groups. (b) Change of cocaine-abstinent rates per week by treatment groups. (c) Fitted probability of presenting any cocaine-free urine per week among the different treatment groups. This is calculated from mixed-effect ordinal regression analysis models that controlled for the baseline cocaine-free urines and that included years of cocaine and heroin use as covariates. Difference between tiagabine and gabapentin groups ($Z = -2.48$, d.f. = 1, $p = 0.01$). Difference between tiagabine and placebo groups ($Z = 3.90$, d.f. = 1, $p = 0.0001$).

Reprinted from *Drug and Alcohol Dependence*, 87, Gonzalez, G., Desai, R., Sofuoglu, et al. Clinical efficacy of gabapentin versus tiagabine for reducing cocaine use among cocaine dependent methadone-treated patients, pp. 1–9. Copyright (2007), with permission from Elsevier.

Topiramate is an anti-epileptic that is thought to act as an agonist at GABA_A receptors. Research has additionally demonstrated its potential clinical efficacy in substance addiction. Long-term outcomes for alcohol abstinence appear to be better for topiramate compared to placebo treatment (see Figure 8.9). Topiramate also significantly increases cocaine abstinence compared to placebo, suggesting a potential clinical effect in cocaine-dependent populations.

Vigabatrin (γ-vinyl GABA) is an anti-epileptic. Vigabatrin irreversibly inhibits GABA-transaminase (GABA-T), the principal enzyme responsible for the

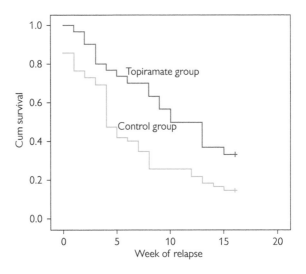

Figure 8.9 Topiramate increases abstinence from alcohol. The cumulative probability function of reaching 16 weeks of abstinence by group. Although 67 patients in total (78.8%) had relapsed to alcohol use by the end of the study (16 weeks after discharge), relapse rate was significantly lower in the topiramate group (66.7%) compared with the control group (85.5%) (p <0.05). Also, median duration of abstinence in the topiramate group was significantly longer compared to the non-medicated group (10 weeks vs 4 weeks; log rank test, p <0.01). Cox proportional hazard model showed that risk of relapse was 56% lower among patients receiving topiramate compared to controls (HR = 0.515, 95% CI: 0.304–0.874, p <0.05).

breakdown of synaptic GABA. Vigabatrin has been shown to rapidly elevate GABA concentrations in humans. Vigabatrin blocks cocaine-induced dopamine release in the VS and appears to prevent the behavioural manifestations of cocaine dependence in animals. Compared to placebo, vigabatrin has been shown to increase rates of abstinence in cocaine-dependent volunteers (Brodie at al. 2009). While vigabatrin has not proved efficacious in attenuating the positive subjective effects of methamphetamine in the laboratory, its use in promoting methamphetamine abstinence has yet to be tested.

8.4 Conclusion

GABA is the major inhibitory neurotransmitter in the brain. GABAergic interneurons and GABA projection neurons are located in dopamine midbrain and striatal regions. These regions are important in the reinforcing effects of substances of abuse. GABA is exploited by substances of abuse, such as alcohol and benzodiazepines, which may result in a downregulation of the GABA system. Stimulants, however, may sensitize the GABA system. Therefore, the chronic abuse of substances may alter the balance of GABA functioning. Disturbances in the GABA system, however, may pre-date substance abuse and addiction.

Medications that boost the availability of GABA or mimic its effects at receptors may possess some clinical potential with respect to abstinence or in attenuating the acute reinforcing effects of substances. Attenuating the reinforcing effects of substances may reduce their use. GABAergic compounds, such as benzodiazepines, significantly interact with certain opioid medications to increase their reinforcing and sedative effects, however.

REFERENCES AND FURTHER READING

Addolorato G, Caputo F, Capristo E, et al. (2002). Baclofen efficacy in reducing alcohol craving and intake: a preliminary double-blind randomized controlled study. *Alcohol and Alcoholism*, **37**, 504–8.

Addolorato G, Leggio L, Abenavoli L, et al. (2006). Baclofen in the treatment of alcohol withdrawal syndrome: a comparative study vs diazepam. *American Journal of Medicine*, **119**, 276. e13–18.

Addolorato G, Leggio L, Ferrulli A, et al. (2007). Effectiveness and safety of baclofen for maintenance of alcohol abstinence in alcohol-dependent patients with liver cirrhosis: randomised, double-blind controlled study. *Lancet*, **370**, 1915–22.

Brodie JD, Case BG, Figueroa E, et al. (2009). Randomized, double-blind, placebo-controlled trial of vigabatrin for the treatment of cocaine dependence in Mexican parolees. *American Journal of Psychiatry*, **166**, 1269–77.

Chick J and Nutt DJ (2012). Substitution therapy for alcoholism: time for a reappraisal? *Journal of Psychopharmacology*, **26(2)**, 205–12.

Gonzalez G, Desai R, Sofuoglu M, et al. (2007). Clinical efficacy of gabapentin versus tiagabine for reducing cocaine use among cocaine-dependent methadone-treated patients. *Drug and Alcohol Dependence*, **87**, 1–9.

Lingford-Hughes A, Reid vAG, Myers J, et al. (2010). A [11C]Ro15 4513 PET study suggests that alcohol dependence in man is associated with reduced alpha5 benzodiazepine receptors in limbic regions. *Journal of Psychopharmacology*, **26**, 273–81.

Lintzeris N, Mitchell TB, Bond AJ, et al. (2007). Pharmacodynamics of diazepam co-administered with methadone or buprenorphine under high dose conditions in opioid-dependent patients. *Drug and Alcohol Dependence*, **91**, 187–94.

Paparrigopoulos T, Tzavellas E, Karaiskos D, et al. (2011). Treatment of alcohol dependence with low-dose topiramate: an open-label controlled study. *BMC Psychiatry*, **11**, 41.

Sofuoglu M, Poling J, Mitchell E, et al. (2005). Tiagabine affects the subjective responses to cocaine in humans. *Pharmacology Biochemistry and Behavior*, **82**, 569–73.

Volkow ND, Wang GJ, Fowler JS, et al. (1998). Enhanced sensitivity to benzodiazepines in active cocaine-abusing subjects: a PET study. *American Journal of Psychiatry*, **155**, 200–6.

CHAPTER 8

The glutamate system and addiction

KEY POINTS

- Addiction involves enduring neuroplasticity in the reward circuitry of the brain.
- Neuroplasticity is a result of glutamate-dependent long-term potentiation.
- Glutamate is an excitatory neurotransmitter.
- Glutamate release is involved in alcohol and drug relapse in response to drug cues.
- There are changes in glutamate receptor functioning in substance addiction.
- Medications that reduce glutamate tone may prevent alcohol and drug relapse.

Chronic substance use is thought to induce enduring pathological changes in the brain. One of these changes is a form of synaptic plasticity within neural circuits important for adaptive behavioural responding. This synaptic plasticity, particularly within dopamine midbrain and striatal regions, is dependent upon the excitatory neurotransmitter glutamate. Significantly, evidence points to similar glutamate-dependent processes involved in both learning and memory and in the development of substance addiction.

In this chapter, we will discuss the recruitment of glutamate over dopamine-dependent substrates in addiction and its implication for medications that treat addiction through the modulation of glutamate signalling in the brain.

9.1 The glutamate system

Glutamate is the primary excitatory neurotransmitter in the brain. The main glutamate projection neurons (see Figure 9.1) arise from a number of different nuclei, including the thalamus and prefrontal cortex (PFC). The transamination of α-ketoglutarate within the presynaptic nerve terminals of these nuclei produces glutamate, a small proportion of which is used as a neurotransmitter (most serves a metabolic function). The regions in receipt of these glutamate projection neurons are numerous and are known to include the midbrain ventral tegmental area (VTA) and the striatum.

When released from presynaptic projection neurons, glutamate binds with two types of receptors. These are ionotropic and metabotropic. *N*-methyl-D-aspartate (NMDA), kainate, and α-amino-3-hydroxy-5-methyl-4-isoxazolepropionic acid

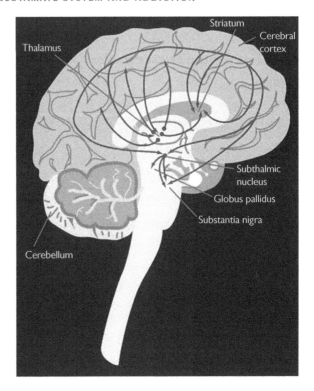

Figure 9.1 Glutamate pathways in the brain. The main pathways are: the cortico-cortical pathways; the pathways between the thalamus and the cortex; and the extrapyramidal pathway (the projections between the cortex and striatum).

(AMPA) receptors are ionotropic: when activated, they open ion channels that pass sodium and/or calcium ions across the neuronal membrane. The G-protein coupled glutamate receptors (mGluR) are metabotropic: when activated, they regulate intracellular adenylyl cyclase and cyclic adenosine monophosphate (cAMP) activity. There are three groups of the mGluR, which make up a total of eight receptor subtypes (mGluR$_{1-8}$). Glutamate can also come from glutamine. When sequestered into nearby astrocytes, glutamate is converted to glutamine via glutamine synthase. Here, glutamine diffuses out of astrocytes and into the nearby nerve terminals where it is converted back into glutamate via glutaminase.

NMDA receptors are thought to play a significant role in the development of addiction. They are located on postsynaptic neurons (see Figure 9.2). Their stimulation is rapidly converted into a postsynaptic electrical signal and is involved in the processes of long-term potentiation (LTP) and long-term depression (LTD).

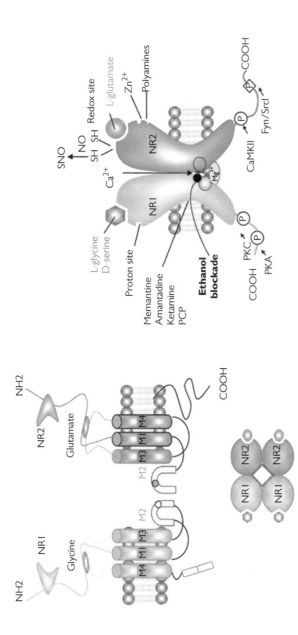

Figure 9.2 The NMDA receptor complex. The principal components of the NMDA receptor. There are binding sites for glycine on the NR1 subunit and glutamate on the NR2 subunit. Both glycine and glutamate must bind to their respective sites to activate the receptor. There are also binding sites for polyamines, magnesium (Mg^{2+}), zinc (Zn^{2+}), and protons. The depolarization of the receptor must be sufficient to remove Mg^{2+} blockade. There are also recognition sites for compounds, such as ketamine and phencyclidine (PCP), which are antagonists at the receptor. Ethanol also blocks the NMDA receptor, which may possibly contribute to NMDA receptor upregulation in alcoholism.

LTP and LTD are long-lasting increases or decreases, respectively, in synaptic transmission. These cellular processes are hypothesized to underlie information storage in the brain as they are rapidly established and strengthened by repetition. NDMA receptors, therefore, are involved in synaptic plasticity—a strengthening of connections between neurons. This is an important neurochemical foundation of learning and memory.

The NMDA receptor has a number of recognition binding sites, including those for phencyclidine, MK-801 (dizocilpine), and ketamine. Alcohol blocks the NMDA receptor (see Figure 9.2). Consequentially, there is an upregulation in NDMA receptor functioning. Features of this upregulation include tolerance to the effects of alcohol as well as increased cortical excitability, withdrawal seizures, and withdrawal-related neurotoxicity. In animals and in humans, drugs that block NMDA glutamate receptors or reduce glutamate release appear to be effective in suppressing the alcohol abstinence syndrome (see 9.4 Treatment).

9.2 Substance addiction—VTA glutamate in the development of addiction

The first indication that glutamate was involved in stimulant addiction came from studies investigating the neurobiology of behavioural sensitization. Behavioural sensitization involves a progressive increase in the motor stimulatory effects of stimulants following their repeated and intermittent administration. Sensitization development has been hypothesized to represent a shift from drug 'liking' to drug 'wanting'. It has also been hypothesized to underlie compulsive substance use in humans.

Behavioural sensitization has been demonstrated for a variety of substances, particularly those acting directly through the dopamine system, such as amphetamines, cocaine, and nicotine. It may potentially model elements of craving and relapse in humans. Antagonists at NMDA receptors in the VTA have been shown to block the development of this behavioural sensitization in animals.

The emergence of behavioural sensitization in response to substances of addiction is thought to involve glutamate-dependent LTP at NMDA receptors on dopamine neurons in the VTA. For example, a single exposure to cocaine has been found to potentiate excitatory synapses in the VTA, which is dependent upon NMDA receptors. In addition, enhanced synaptic transmission occurs via an increase in the number (or function) of postsynaptic AMPA receptors. This finding has also been shown for the development of drug self-administration in animals.

While it is less clear which glutamatergic afferents to the VTA are critical for the development of addiction, the role of glutamate-dependent LTP in the VTA appears to suggest that synaptic plasticity in midbrain dopamine neurons is essential. During repeated drug administration, neuroplasticity is also taking place in the PFC. Glutamate neurons in the PFC appear to be sensitized by substances, such as psychostimulants. This may be commensurate with the exaggerated release of glutamate in the ventral striatum (VS) during drug-seeking, as described in 9.3 Substance addiction.

9.3 Substance addiction—nucleus accumbens (NAcc) glutamate in the expression of addiction

There also appears to be a role for glutamate in the expression of addiction behaviour, particularly in the NAcc region of the VS. The reinstatement model of drug-seeking has been used extensively to examine the expression of addiction-related behaviour in animals. This model has also demonstrated a preferential role for the core region of NAcc (as opposed to the shell) in the expression of reinstatement. As described in Chapter 4, there are discrete hedonic 'hotspots' for substance 'liking', one of which is in the shell of the NAcc. Animals will learn to self-administer dopaminergic drugs (e.g. cocaine, D1R/D2R receptor agonists) more into the shell of the NAcc than the core. This may suggest that there are differential roles for the shell and core in substance 'liking' and 'wanting', respectively, the latter of which may occur following chronic substance use and which may be important for substance use reinstatement (i.e. relapse).

During the reinstatement model, animals will typically self-administer a drug (e.g. cocaine) under operant conditions for prolonged periods of time. This operant responding for the drug is intended to mimic chronic drug self-administration in humans. Following this chronic drug self-administration period, animals will then undergo extinction training—responding on the previous reinforced (i.e. active) operandum will no longer elicit primary reinforcement (i.e. drug delivery). This extinction training will gradually lead to a significant reduction in the level of responding on the drug-paired operandum. Following extinction, a conditioned cue, drug-priming injection, or a stressor will be introduced to trigger the reinstatement of drug-seeking behaviour—as indexed by a renewed increase in responding on the previously drug-paired operandum. The reinstatement of increased responding is thought to model relapse in humans.

The reinstatement of cocaine-seeking is associated with increased glutamate release into the core of the NAcc. Moreover, AMPA receptor blockade in the core prevents the reinstatement of responding to a drug or cue prime. The inhibition of glutamate PFC afferents into this region attenuates drug-seeking induced by cocaine, heroin, stress, and cues. The inhibition of amygdala glutamate afferents also blocks cue and heroin reinstatement in animals.

In addition to enhanced glutamate transmission in the NAcc core during the expression of drug-seeking or sensitization, there are also a number of glutamate-related cellular adaptations produced by chronic psychostimulant administration. Research points towards augmented AMPA sensitivity—AMPA stimulation induces motor activity or the reinstatement of drug-seeking.

9.4 Treatment—regulating glutamate release for attenuating addiction behaviours

Given the apparent role of glutamate in regulating both the development and expression of addictive behaviours in animal models, glutamate may be a potential pharmacotherapeutic target for substance addiction in humans. Figure 9.3 illustrates the putative glutamatergic mechanisms of action of eight anti-addiction medications. While these medications have very contrasting pharmacological mechanisms of action (that are not all specific to glutamate) their overall effect is to reduce glutamate tone in the brain.

The regulation of non-synaptic glial glutamate release by stimulating cystine-glutamate exchange (see xc– in the N-acetylcysteine section of Figure 9.3) has recently come to light as a potential medication target. xc– is involved in exchanging the uptake of one cystine in exchange for the release of one molecule of intracellular glutamate into the extracellular space. Cocaine self-administration in animals has been shown to downregulate the cystine–glutamate exchanger. Therefore, restoring the functional integrity of this exchanger may possess some efficacy in reducing substance use by increasing synaptic glutamate at mGluR2/3 regulating autoreceptors—thus reducing glutamate tone.

N-acetylcysteine (NAC) is an xc– agonist that has been shown to indirectly stimulate mGluR2/3 to reduce glutamate release in the NAcc and inhibit cocaine-seeking in animals (Amen et al. 2011). In parallel, preliminary clinical research indicates that repeated administration (4 days) of NAC (1200–2400 mg/day) in cocaine-dependent subjects produces a significant reduction in craving following acute cocaine (Amen et al. 2011).

NAC has also been shown to reduce cocaine-related withdrawal symptoms and craving (LaRowe et al. 2006). Cocaine use was either terminated or significantly reduced over a four week trial using NAC in cocaine abusers. NAC has also been shown to significantly reduce glutamate levels in the dorsal anterior cingulate of cocaine-dependent subjects (Schmaal et al. 2012). This may lend credence to the supposition that NAC-induced reductions in glutamate tone are involved in the clinical efficacy of this compound.

Other compounds that influence glutamate functioning may also possess some efficacy. **Acamprosate** (see Figure 9.3) is an NMDA antagonist (and possibly a GABA$_A$ receptor agonist). It has some clinical potential in alcohol dependence. Theories posit that acamprosate may restore an imbalance between excitatory and inhibitory neurotransmission that results from chronic alcohol consumption. Indeed, a recent study in detoxified alcoholics has shown that four weeks of acamprosate treatment significantly reduces glutamate in the anterior cingulate gyrus (Umhau et al. 2010). The overall bio-availability of acamprosate, however, remains poor (i.e. <20%) and requires doses in the range of 2–3 g per day in order to demonstrate clinical efficacy. The requirement for three doses per day, therefore, may act as a compliance barrier in some patients.

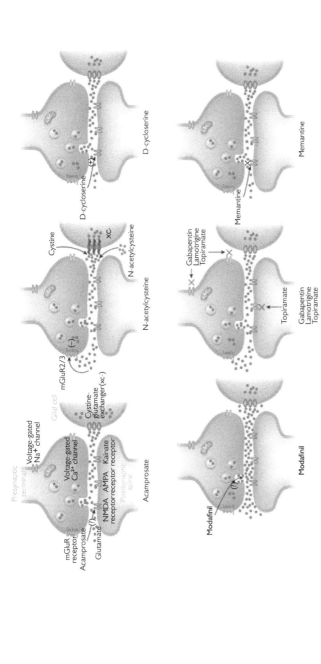

Figure 9.3 Glutamatergic mechanisms of action of anti-addiction medications. Acamprosate modulates the activity of NMDA receptors. N-acetylcysteine (NAC) stimulates the cystine-glutamate exchanger (xc–) on glia to normalize extracellular levels of glutamate. D-cycloserine (DCS) is a partial agonist at the glycine co-agonist binding site. Modafinil increases extracellular levels of glutamate in various brain regions. Gabapentin, lamotrigine, topiramate are anticonvulsants that reduce the release of glutamate by blocking Na$^+$ and Ca^{2+} influx. Topiramate has the unique ability to also antagonize GluR5-containing AMPA receptors. Memantine is a non-competitive NMDA receptor antagonist.

Reprinted from *Pharmacology Biochemistry and Behavior*, 100, Olive, M. F., Cleva, R. M., Kalivas, P. W., & Malcolm, R. J., Glutamatergic medications for the treatment of drug and behavioral addictions. pp. 801–810. Copyright (2012), with permission from Elsevier.

The partial NMDA agonist **D-cycloserine** (DCS—see Figure 9.2) has also been tested. DCS mimics the actions of glycine at the glycine$_B$ receptor. Both glycine and glutamate are necessary for NMDA receptor functioning (see Figure 9.1). NMDA receptor functioning is known to be blunted in alcohol-dependent patients, appearing to support the hypothesis that NMDA receptor upregulation increases tolerance to the effects of alcohol. DCS has been shown to reduce cocaine-induced conditioned place preference in animals. It has proved less favourable in cocaine-dependent humans—it actually increases cue-induced relapse. In alcoholics, it has shown some promise, but the wide range of craving responses in alcoholics precludes any firm conclusion regarding its potential clinical efficacy.

Gabapentin (see Figure 9.2) is an anticonvulsant medication. It has a general inhibitory effect on neuronal transmission by inhibiting presynaptic voltage-gated Na^+ and Ca^{2+} channels. As a result, gabapentin inhibits the release of various neurotransmitters, including glutamate. Gabapentin may be efficacious in alleviating the somatic symptoms of alcohol withdrawal. Gabapentin (600–1500 mg/day) reduces alcohol and cocaine craving. It does not appear to reduce methamphetamine use.

Lamotrigine (see Figure 9.2) has a similar mechanism of action to gabapentin. Lamotrigine inhibits the somatic signs of alcohol withdrawal and craving for alcohol. Likewise, it may possess some efficacy for reducing cocaine use and craving but not the subjective effects of cocaine. **Topiramate** (see Figure 9.2), while similar to gabapentin and lamotrigine, is also an antagonist at AMPA receptors containing the GluR5 subunit. In addition to the attenuation of alcohol withdrawal symptoms, it may also attenuate alcohol's subjective effects, alcohol craving, and heavy consumption in alcoholic patients. It may even be superior to naltrexone in preventing alcohol relapse. It has been shown to reduce cocaine use and craving in cocaine-dependent individuals. Typical effective doses range from 75 to 350 mg/day.

Modafinil (see Figure 9.2), while an inhibitor of the dopamine transporter, has also been shown to elevate extracellular levels of glutamate in numerous brain regions, including the dorsal striatum. The potential efficacy of modafinil in substance addiction has already been addressed with respect to dopamine. Clinically effective doses of modafinil are typically in the range of 200–400 mg/day.

Finally, **memantine** (see Figure 9.2) is a non-competitive NMDA receptor antagonist. It is also an antagonist at the serotonin 3 receptor (5-HT$_3$) and at nicotinic acetylcholine receptors. Memantine has shown some efficacy in reducing withdrawal symptoms in detoxifying alcoholics and opiate addicts and is superior to placebo in attenuating ongoing drinking and/or craving for alcohol in alcoholics. It has been suggested that the attenuation of craving for alcohol may be a result of the alcohol-like subjective effects of memantine. Typical doses are 30–60 mg/day range.

9.5 Conclusion

Substance abuse induces neuroplasticity within midbrain, striatal, and PFC circuitry. Heightened neural activity in the PFC-NAcc pathway appears to accompany this neuroplasticity. Neuroplasticity is highly dependent upon the excitatory neurotransmitter glutamate at NMDA receptors. The neuroplasticity within this circuitry is sustained during substance abstinence and may provide a neural substrate for a vulnerability to relapse in substance addiction.

Medications that possess the efficacy to reduce glutamate tone in the PFC-NAcc pathway may reduce craving and, ultimately, relapse in substance dependence. At this time, however, there is still a scarcity of preclinical and clinical data in humans demonstrating the unequivocal efficacy of these medications. Further research is required to show how the modulation of glutamate transmission in the brain confers clinical benefits in substance addiction.

REFERENCES AND FURTHER READING

Amen SL, Piacentine LB, Ahmad ME, et al. (2011). Repeated N-acetyl cysteine reduces cocaine seeking in rodents and craving in cocaine-dependent humans. *Neuropsychopharmacology*, **36**, 871–78.

Baker DA, McFarland K, Lake RW, et al. (2003). Neuroadaptations in cystine-glutamate exchange underlie cocaine relapse. *Nature Neuroscience*, **6**, 743–49.

Glue P and Nutt D (1990). Overexcitement and disinhibition. Dynamic neurotransmitter interactions in alcohol withdrawal. *British Journal of Psychiatry*, **157**, 491–9.

Krystal JH, Petrakis IL, Limoncelli D, et al. (2011). Characterization of the interactive effects of glycine and D-cycloserine in men: further evidence for enhanced NMDA receptor function associated with human alcohol dependence. *Neuropsychopharmacology*, **36**, 701–10.

LaRowe SD, Mardikian P, Malcolm R, et al. (2006). Safety and tolerability of N-acetylcysteine in cocaine-dependent individuals. *American Journal on Addictions*, **15**, 105–10.

Mardikian PN, LaRowe SD, Hedden S, et al. (2007). An open-label trial of N-acetylcysteine for the treatment of cocaine dependence: a pilot study. *Progress in Neuropsychopharmacology & Biological Psychiatry*, **31**, 389–94.

Olive MF, Cleva RM, Kalivas PW, et al. (2012). Glutamatergic medications for the treatment of drug and behavioral addictions. *Pharmacology, Biochemistry and Behavior*, **100**, 801–10.

Schmaal L, Veltman DJ, Nederveen A, et al. (2012). N-acetylcysteine normalizes glutamate levels in cocaine-dependent patients: a randomized crossover magnetic resonance spectroscopy study. *Neuropsychopharmacology*, **37**, 2143–52.

Umhau JC, Momenan R, Schwandt ML, et al. (2010). Effect of acamprosate on magnetic resonance spectroscopy measures of central glutamate in detoxified alcohol-dependent individuals: a randomized controlled experimental medicine study. *Archives of General Psychiatry*, **67**, 1069–77.

Watson BJ, Wilson S, Griffin L, et al. (2011). A pilot study of the effectiveness of D-cycloserine during cue-exposure therapy in abstinent alcohol-dependent subjects. *Psychopharmacology (Berl)*, **216**, 121–9.

The opioid system and addiction

KEY POINTS

- The brain contains a complex system of endogenous opioid peptides.
- These peptides are called endorphins, encephalins, and dynorphin.
- Endorphins preferentially bind to the mu opioid receptor (mOR).
- Encephalins preferentially bind to the delta receptor (dOR).
- Dynorphin preferentially binds to the kappa receptor (kOR).
- Opiates, such as heroin and morphine, also stimulate the mOR.
- The mOR is upregulated in substance addiction.
- Genetic polymorphisms at the mOR influence subjective responses to alcohol.

The opioid system of the brain is the major target for opiate drugs, such as morphine and heroin, and has been implicated in processes, such as pain, stress, and reward. Recent findings from human brain imaging research, however, are beginning to suggest that substance addiction per se may be associated with alterations in this system. These alterations may influence the craving, distress, and dysphoria found in early alcohol and drug abstinence.

In this chapter, we will discuss the brain opioid system and its neuropharmacology and specifically examine the effects of substance abuse on the endorphin system. The implications for treatment will also be discussed.

10.1 The opioid system

Opiate substances of addiction, such as heroin, reduce anxiety and decrease sensitivity to stimuli while inducing euphoria and sedation. They mimic the effects of endogenous substances on a variety of opioid receptor subtypes in the brain. These are the mu, kappa, and delta opioid receptor (mOR/kOR/dOR) subtypes. These are G-protein receptors that are negatively coupled to adenylyl cyclase. Their stimulation, therefore, results in reduced neuronal intracellular signalling.

There are a number of endogenous substances which produce different effects at these receptors. The endogenous opioid peptide β-endorphin preferentially binds with the mOR. Opiate substances of abuse also act at the mOR subtype, and this underlies their reinforcing effects and abuse potential. For example, antagonists, such as naltrexone, block heroin reinforcement, with mOR 'knock-out' mice unwilling to self-administer heroin. The mOR is located in a variety of brain regions, including the orbitofrontal cortex (OFC), thalamus, hippocampus, locus coeruleus, midbrain ventral tegmental area (VTA), nucleus accumbens (NAcc)/ ventral striatum (VS), and amygdala.

Opiates mediate their reinforcing effects directly in the NAcc at the mOR. Opiates also produce their reinforcing effects indirectly. This indirect mechanism of action is through mOR inhibition of GABA functioning in the VTA. The binding of opiates to the mOR disinhibits dopamine VTA projections to the NAcc (see Figure 10.1).

The endogenous opioid system, and particularly the mOR, interfaces with environmental events, both positive (e.g. relevant emotional stimuli) and negative (e.g. stressors). Significantly, research has demonstrated that individuals reporting high impulsiveness have significantly higher regional mOR concentrations in a number of brain regions, including the OFC, NAcc, and amygdala. This may suggest that higher mOR numbers, in brain regions complicit in motivation and reward learning, bestow a greater vulnerability for impulsive/risky behaviours, such as substance abuse.

Encephalin peptides (i.e. met and leu encephalin) preferentially bind to the dOR. The dOR subtype is located at its highest densities in the NAcc, caudate,

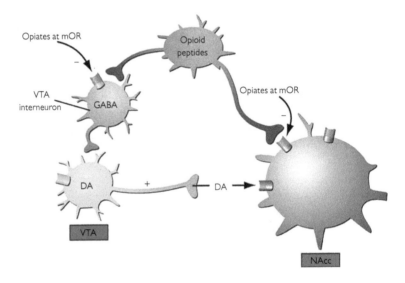

Figure 10.1 Pharmacology of opiate substances of abuse, such as heroin or morphine. Opiates disinhibit dopamine VTA projections to the NAcc. Indirectly, they inhibit GABAergic interneurons in the VTA, which disinhibits VTA dopamine neurons to the NAcc. Opiates also directly act on opioid receptors on NAcc neurons.

putamen, and cerebral cortex. They are located on presynaptic nerve terminals where they inhibit the release of other neurotransmitters (e.g. dopamine).

The dynorphin peptide preferentially binds to the kOR. The kOR is located in the hypothalamus and striatum (i.e. NAcc, caudate, and putamen). The binding of opiates or dynorphin to the kOR is thought to induce the dysphoric effects of these substances. This may be due to kOR ligands inhibiting the release of dopamine in the striatum. Interestingly, substances of abuse have been shown to increase the release of dynorphin in this region. This may implicate the dynorphin system in the reported dysphoria many substance abusers report following chronic consumption.

10.2 Substance addiction

Several studies to-date appear to suggest that the brain opioid system is activated by substances of abuse. For example, a high dose of amphetamine (i.e. indirect dopamine agonist) has been shown to reduce carfentanil (mOR agonist) binding in a number of regions, including the frontal cortex, putamen, and insula (see Figure 10.2). This effect is due to amphetamine-induced release of endorphins that displace the PET radioligand 11C-carfentanil. This effect has also been shown for alcohol in the OFC and NAcc of both control subjects and heavy drinkers (see Figure 10.3).

Also, the administration of naltrexone, an opioid receptor antagonist, in healthy human volunteers has been shown to attenuate the acute, positive effects of substances of abuse, such as amphetamine and alcohol, that do not directly act at the mOR. These results suggest that there are robust interactions between dopamine and opioid mechanisms in the brain. This further indicates that the chronic use and abuse of addictive substances is likely to have enduring effects on the opioid system.

Research suggests that the early stages of abstinence may be associated with alterations to the endorphin system in substance addiction. The OFC is involved in the processes of motivation and drive for rewards and the attribution of salience to reinforcing stimuli. Increased mOR binding in this region has been shown to predict time to relapse in cocaine addicts (Gorelick et al. 2008). The upregulation of the mOR in the OFC may enhance the motivation to use cocaine during abstinence—it may be a biomarker of relapse risk in substance addiction.

The endogenous opioid system may also play a significant role in alcohol dependence. In early abstinent alcoholics, there are elevated mOR numbers (indexed by increased carfentanil binding), compared to healthy controls in several regions implicated in addiction, including the striatum and amygdala (Weers et al. 2011). This suggests a possible upregulation of the mOR and/or a reduction in endogenous opioid peptide release following chronic alcohol use.

Projections from the VTA to VS are, in part, responsible for initiating the motivation for rewards. The initial weeks of alcohol abstinence have provided evidence for greater mOR availability in the VS compared to healthy controls. The higher

○ Putamen
○ Insula
○ Frontal cortex

Figure 10.2 **Amphetamines release endorphins.** Regions in healthy volunteers where a high dose of amphetamine displaced the mOR agonist carfentanil significantly more than a low dose of amphetamine.

Reprinted from *Biological Psychiatry*, 72, Colasanti, A., Searle, G. E., Long, C. J. et al. Endogenous opioid release in the human brain reward system induced by acute amphetamine administration, pp. 371–377. Copyright (2012), Society of Biological Psychiatry. Published by Elsevier Inc.

availability of the mOR in this region is also significantly correlated with the intensity of alcohol craving (Heinz et al. 2005). This may suggest that greater mOR numbers in this region predict a greater vulnerability for relapse in early alcohol abstinence.

Striatal dopamine is involved in substance reward, and alcohol has been shown to induce dopamine release in this region in humans. Humans vary substantially in their responses to alcohol, however. This variability may be related to a genetic susceptibility for alcohol-use disorders—genetics are thought to account for more than half the disease risk in this condition. Importantly, a functional variation in the mOR may contribute to this variation by modulating alcohol-induced dopamine release.

Significantly, it has been shown that a functional *OPRM1* A118G polymorphism influences striatal dopamine responses to alcohol in social drinkers (see Figure 10.4). The A118G polymorphism of the *OPRM1* gene has been shown to confer functional differences to the mOR, such that the G variant binds β-endorphin three times more strongly than the A variant. It has also been shown that individuals

Figure 10.3 Alcohol releases endorphins. Changes in mOR binding in ROIs following alcohol consumption. Top panel of the figures shows spatially co-registered coronal MRI (left) and PET (right) images from a single representative control subject, indicating designation of individually drawn NAcc ROIs. Left: a coronal section MRI with the NAcc ROI hand-drawn in orange. Right: carfentanil binding potential, with highest binding potential in hot colours (see colour scale). The bar graph shows the binding potential (B_{max}/K_d) NAcc ROI. **p <0.01, on paired t-tests for heavy drinking (n = 12) and control subjects (n = 13) before and after alcohol consumption.

Figure 10.4 mOR genetics predict striatal dopamine responses to alcohol. Human PET study. Axial view of group maps, showing change of [¹¹C]-raclopride binding potential (ΔBP; nCi/cc) between placebo and alcohol sessions in (A) AA individuals and (B) AG individuals. Colour bars indicate corresponding ΔBP values. Reduction in raclopride binding is attributed to competition with dopamine released by the alcohol challenge; thus, a negative ΔBP indicates an increase in endogenous dopamine release. (C) Relative change in binding potential (% Δ BP) for [¹¹C]-raclopride between alcohol and placebo sessions in four striatal regions of interest. Data are least square means (± SEM). Main genotype effect: $p = 0.006$; *$p < 0.05$ on post hoc tests within individual regions. AVS, anterior ventral striatum; PVS, posterior ventral striatum. (D) Schematic of PET sessions and blood alcohol concentration profiles over time during the alcohol session (mean ± SEM). There was no significant difference between genotypes ($F[1,24] = 0.51$, $p = 0.48$).

Reprinted by permission from Macmillan Publishers Ltd: *Molecular Psychiatry*, 16, 8, Ramchandani, V. A., Umhau, J., Pavon F.J. et al., A genetic determinant of the striatal dopamine response to alcohol in men, pp. 809–817. Copyright © 2010, Rights Managed by Nature Publishing Group.

with the G allele report higher subjective feelings of intoxication, stimulation, sedation, and happiness in response to alcohol, compared to individuals with the A allele.

10.3 Treatment

Clinical trials have focussed on mOR blockade with naltrexone in substance dependence. Naltrexone, acamprosate (NMDA antagonist and GABA$_A$ agonist), and their combination appear significantly more effective than placebo in preventing alcohol relapse (Kiefer et al. 2003). Naltrexone has also shown some promise for the treatment of amphetamine dependence. Reduced craving levels and the consumption of amphetamine have been shown during naltrexone, compared to placebo. Depot injections of naltrexone have also been found to increase treatment retention in heroin addiction.

Both naltrexone and nalmefene (an mOR antagonist and a partial kOR agonist) have been shown to reduce alcohol use in alcoholics. This has been shown using a choice consumption paradigm following a standard 'priming' alcohol dose in a bar-laboratory setting (see Figure 10.5).

The efficacy of naltrexone in the treatment and management of alcoholism may also be moderated by genetics. The A118G polymorphism of the *OPRM1* gene has been shown to confer differences in how people respond to the efficacy of naltrexone in attenuating the reinforcing effects of alcohol. In individuals with, at least, one copy of the G allele, effects of naltrexone on blunting alcohol-induced 'high' were significantly stronger (Ray and Hutchison 2007).

10.4 Conclusion

There is strong evidence for dopamine–endorphin interactions in the brain. The mOR findings in addiction may endorse this neuroadaptation as an important neural biomarker of early abstinence and relapse risk. There is also evidence for the effects of genetic polymorphisms at the mOR—effects that confer a greater dopamine response to the reinforcing effects of alcohol. There is evidence for the potential efficacy of mOR antagonists in reducing relapse, increasing treatment retention, and attenuating the subjective effects of substances of abuse. The effects of antagonists at the mOR may also be genetically moderated, suggesting that only some individuals will show a clinical response to these compounds. Medications with partial agonist activity at the kOR, such as nalmefene, may confer an additional clinical advantage—reduce binging following relapse in substance dependence.

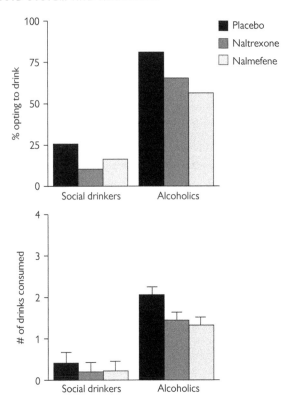

Figure 10.5 mOR blockade reduces drinking. Percentage of subjects in each medication group opting to drink during the free-drinking period (top panel) and the average number of drinks (± SEM) consumed during this period (bottom panel).

Reprinted by permission from Macmillan Publishers Ltd: *Neuropsychopharmacology*, 28, 4, Drobes, D. J., Anton R. F., Thoma, S.E. et al., A clinical laboratory paradigm for evaluating medication effects on alcohol consumption: naltrexone and nalmefene, pp. 755–764. Copyright © 2003, Rights Managed by Nature Publishing Group.

REFERENCES AND FURTHER READING

Colasanti A, Searle GE, Long CJ, et al. (2012). Endogenous opioid release in the human brain reward system induced by acute amphetamine administration. *Biological Psychiatry*, **72**, 371–7.

Comer SD, Sullivan MA, Yu E, et al. (2006). Injectable, sustained-release naltrexone for the treatment of opioid dependence: a randomized, placebo-controlled trial. *Archives of General Psychiatry*, **63**, 210–18.

Drobes DJ, Anton RF, Thomas SE, et al. (2003). A clinical laboratory paradigm for evaluating medication effects on alcohol consumption: naltrexone and nalmefene. *Neuropsychopharmacology*, **28**, 755–64.

Gianoulakis C (2009). Endogenous opioids and addiction to alcohol and other drugs of abuse. *Current Topics in Medicinal Chemistry*, **9**(11), 999–1015.

Gorelick DA, Kim YK, Bencherif B, et al. (2008). Brain mu opioid receptor binding: relationship to relapse to cocaine use after monitored abstinence. *Psychopharmacology (Berl)*, **200**, 475–86.

Heinz A, Reimold M, Wrase J, et al. (2005). Correlation of stable elevations in striatal mu opioid receptor availability in detoxified alcoholic patients with alcohol craving: a positron emission tomography study using carbon 11-labeled carfentanil. *Archives of General Psychiatry*, **62**, 57–64.

Jayaram-Lindstrom N, Hammarberg A, Beck O, et al. (2008). Naltrexone for the treatment of amphetamine dependence: a randomized, placebo-controlled trial. *American Journal of Psychiatry*, **165**, 1442–8.

Jayaram-Lindstrom N, Konstenius M, Eksborg S, et al. (2008). Naltrexone attenuates the subjective effects of amphetamine in patients with amphetamine dependence. *Neuropsychopharmacology*, **33**, 1856–63.

Karhuvaara S, Simojoki K, Virta A, et al. (2007). Targeted nalmefene with simple medical management in the treatment of heavy drinkers: a randomized double-blind placebo-controlled multicenter study. *Alcoholism: Clinical and Experimental Research*, **31**(7), 1179–87.

Kiefer F, Jahn H, Tarnaske T, et al. (2003). Comparing and combining naltrexone and acamprosate in relapse prevention of alcoholism: a double-blind, placebo-controlled study. *Archives of General Psychiatry*, **60**(1), 92–9.

Love TM, Stohler CS, and Zubieta JK (2009). Positron emission tomography measures of endogenous opioid neurotransmission and impulsiveness traits in humans. *Archives of General Psychiatry*, **66**, 1124–34.

Mitchell JM, O'Neil JP, Janabi M, et al. (2012). Alcohol consumption induces endogenous opioid release in the human orbitofrontal cortex and nucleus accumbens. *Science Translational Medicine*, **4**, 116ra116.

Ramchandani VA, Umhau J, Pavon FJ, et al. (2010). A genetic determinant of the striatal dopamine response to alcohol in men. *Molecular Psychiatry*, **16**, 809–17.

Ray LA and Hutchison KE (2007). Effects of naltrexone on alcohol sensitivity and genetic moderators of medication response: a double-blind placebo-controlled study. *Archives of General Psychiatry*, **64**, 1069–77.

Weerts EM, Wand GS, Kuwabara H, et al. (2011). Positron emission tomography imaging of mu and delta opioid receptor binding in alcohol-dependent and healthy control subjects. *Alcoholism: Clinical and Experimental Research*, **35**, 2162–73.

CHAPTER 11

Nicotine addiction

KEY POINTS

- Nicotine is a stimulant that is the main psychoactive element of cigarettes.
- Nicotine is an agonist at nicotinic acetylcholine receptors in the brain.
- Nicotine in smoked tobacco is addictive.
- Nicotine causes disturbances to reward and cognitive processing.
- Cigarette smoking presents considerable health risks.
- Cigarette smoking induces high costs on healthcare resources.
- Smoking cessation medications and safer nicotine products (e.g. e-cigs) are now available to treat nicotine addiction.

11.1 Nicotine

The number of cigarette smokers worldwide is estimated at 1.3 billion, although there has been an observed decline in the prevalence of smoking in the developed world. Despite some success in reversing the tobacco epidemic in the developed world, tobacco use continues to increase in less developed countries where insufficient resources and education concerning tobacco use lead to its widespread consumption. Furthermore, it has been estimated, based on current trends of tobacco use, that 70% of the global deaths from tobacco consumption by 2025 will have occurred in developing nations. Despite these statistics and the well-documented health consequences it is extraordinary that people continue to consume tobacco. This continued use in the face of adversity is a sad, but powerful testimony to the effects of nicotine dependence, clearly demonstrating its addictive properties. While the majority of cigarette smokers endorse the desire to quit, reported abstinence rates after 12 months are in the modest region of 5–17%, with the vast majority relapsing to smoking within a week of cessation. Because cigarette smoking presents a considerable health risk and induces high costs on healthcare resources there is a pressing need to understand, in greater detail, the effects of nicotine addiction in the brain, and how changes in functioning may contribute to its continued use.

11.1.1 Nicotine effects

Nicotine exerts its effects within the brain by acting at nicotinic acetylcholine receptors (nAChRs), to mimic the effects of the natural neurotransmitter acetylcholine (ACh). These receptors control cation-selective, ligand-gated channels.

nAChRs are pentameric combinations of 12 genetically distinct homologous subunits ($\alpha2$–$\alpha10$ and $\beta2$–$\beta4$), with each nAChR assumed to be hetero-oligomeric (i.e. composed from various combinations of α and β subunits). Early nicotine binding studies identified two distinct nicotine binding sites in the form of the high affinity $\alpha4\beta2$ and the low affinity $\alpha7$ receptor subtypes, which have subsequently provided evidence concerning structural and functional changes related to nicotine use in the brain (see Figure 11.1).

The release of ACh onto nAChRs throughout the brain takes place through a series of cholinergic forebrain projections, which include the nucleus basalis of

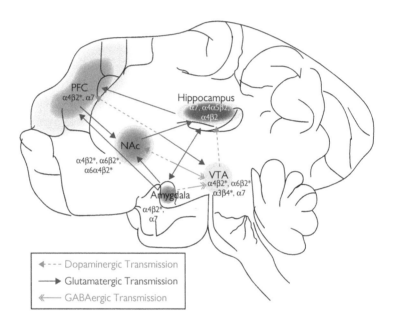

Figure 11.1 Neuronal nicotinic acetylcholine receptors (nAChRs) are widely distributed in different brain regions that include the ventral tegmental area (VTA), nucleus accumbens (NAc), hippocampus, prefrontal cortex (PFC), and amygdala. Activation of nAChRs in these brain areas significantly contributes to the rewarding effects of nicotine. GABAergic (red), glutamatergic (green), and dopaminergic (blue) connections between these structures constitute a major neural circuitry underlying addictive disorders, which includes nicotine addiction.

Meynert (NBM); the diagonal band nucleus; nucleus ansa lenticularis, and part of the magnocellular preoptic nucleus. Approximately two-thirds of the NBM neurons projecting to the cortex are cholinergic, with ~30% GABAergic, which preferentially connect with GABAergic interneurons. nAChRs have been shown to modulate presynaptic glutamate release with further observations of nicotine-induced GABA modulation in multiple brain regions such as the ventral tegmental area (VTA), thalamus, cerebral cortex, and hippocampus. There are also a number of neurotransmitters, which interfere with cortical ACh release, such as dopamine (DA) acting at the NBM, serotonin modulating neuronal activity at the NBM and the release of ACh in the cortex, and norepinephrine, acting as a tonic inhibitor of cortical ACh release. Therefore, the neuroanatomical distribution of nAChRs is likely to contribute to the long-term effects of nicotine administration during chronic smoking—particularly on neuronal networks which contribute to reward processing and cognitive control.

Nicotine, like other stimulant drugs of abuse, activates the mesocorticolimbic DA system. The ventral striatum (VS) has been implicated in the development of nicotine addiction due to its role in processing the hedonic effects of nicotine. Studies using rats, for example, have demonstrated that nicotine stimulates DA neurons in the midbrain VTA, resulting in increased burst firing at the shell of the NAcc. As described in Chapter 4, there are discrete hedonic 'hotspots' for substance 'liking', one of which is in the shell of the NAcc. Animals will learn to self-administer dopaminergic drugs (e.g. amphetamine, cocaine) into the shell of the NAcc. Likewise, nicotine induces DA release in humans. One of the most seminal studies to demonstrate this was conducted by Brody and colleagues (2004). This study showed that in smokers, DA release was significantly increased in striatal regions of the brain following cigarette smoking, compared to smokers who were not allowed to smoke. Significantly, this study also showed that the magnitude of DA release in those who smoked was significantly associated with changes in smoking urges, indicating that nicotine-induced DA release attenuates craving. There is also evidence to suggest that genetic variance within the DA system may explain a significant proportion of the interindividual variability in smoking-induced DA release, suggesting a genetic predisposition to the rewarding effects of nicotine. Smokers with genes associated with low resting DA tone, for example, elicit greater smoking-induced (i.e. phasic) DA release compared with smokers with alternate genotypes (Brody et al. 2006b). These results regarding the effects of nicotine-induced DA release (and particularly in attenuation of craving) support the development of medications for nicotine dependence that modulate DA tone to prevent relapse (see 11.4 Treatments).

Most studies concerning the reinforcing effects of nicotine, however, only use acute administration procedures. Because smoking is a chronic form of behaviour that most likely leads to long-term adaptations in the brain, knowledge concerning changes related to its prolonged use is essential for developing better treatments—particularly treatments that can promote abstinence during the early phases of withdrawal. Indeed, animal studies have documented the long-term effects of nicotine, with research showing a paradoxical up-regulation of α4β2 nAChRs in the brain, perhaps indicating a form of sensitization of the ACh system. Interestingly, striatal DA release is modulated by α4β2 nAChRs in rats, with research showing that chronic nicotine treatment significantly increases α4β2 nAChRs in the VS of monkeys, with a corresponding increase in α4β2 evoked DA release at this region. Given that increased DA neurotransmission in the striatum is also related to self-reported craving in humans, an upregulation of α4β2 nAChRs in striatal regions may be a neurochemical marker for DA-induced craving in nicotine addiction.

Studies in human smokers have shown that smoking saturates α4β2 nAChRs throughout the brain in a dose-dependent manner. Brody and colleagues (2006a), for example, reported that smoking just one to two puffs of a cigarette resulted in 50% occupancy of α4β2 nAChRs for three hours after smoking, and that smoking a full cigarette (or more) resulted in more than 88% receptor occupancy—accompanied by a significant reduction in cigarette craving. This suggests that α4β2 nAChRs play a pivotal role in the effects of cigarette craving in nicotine addiction. Interestingly, Brody and colleagues (2013) has also reported that lesser α4β2 upregulation in human nicotine dependence is associated with a greater likelihood of smoking cessation. Therefore, nicotine induces α4β2 nAChRs adaptations in the brain which are likely to be implicated in disordered reward processing in nicotine addiction, which likely provokes smoking relapse during withdrawal.

11.2 Reward

Disturbances in reward-related brain functioning for non-drug incentives have revealed adaptations in neural circuitry that likely contribute to ongoing smoking behaviour in humans. The reward deficiency syndrome (RDS), for example, views addiction as a deficit in DA motivational circuitry for non-drug incentives such that only substances, such as nicotine, are able to normalize DA. There is evidence to suggest that chronic smokers have DA deficits in the striatum, similar to other addiction populations. Fehr and colleagues (2008), for example, showed that smokers, compared to never smokers, had reduced DA D2/D3 receptor numbers in parts of the striatum, appearing to concur with an RDS view of nicotine addiction. Indeed, these deficits in striatal DA integrity in nicotine addiction are likely to translate into disturbances in reward processing and motivation, particularly during acute abstinence—an effect that provokes relapse. As described in Chapter 4, reward is a central component for driving incentive-based learning, eliciting appropriate responses to stimuli, and the development of goal-directed behaviours. Substances of addiction are conceived to 'hijack' brain circuitry involved in reward by diminishing the motivation value of non-drug rewards while inflating the reward and motivational value of drugs, such as nicotine. This is particularly evident during abstinence in brain regions such as the striatum when deficits in DA functioning are exacerbated by withdrawal, provoking a shift in the bias towards drug incentives. Indeed, Sweitzer and colleagues have elegantly shown that in smokers in early nicotine abstinence (withdrawal), cues that predict potential nicotine (cigarette puffs) elicit greater fMRI activity in striatal and mesocortical brain regions as compared with cues that predict potential monetary rewards. The opposite is observed, however, when smokers are satiated (see Figure 11.2). The results of this study provided the first direct evidence of a dissociated effect of smoking versus non-smoking rewards as a function of nicotine abstinence. This appears to suggest an important neural pathway that may bias the choice to smoke in the presence of alternative, non-drug reinforcement—a substrate involved in smoking relapse. In conclusion, the current, but still limited, literature appears to suggests that chronic smokers (heavily dependent on nicotine) have deficits in striatal DA integrity and reduced striatal non-drug reward-related neural activity, leading one to surmise that there may be nicotine addiction-induced alterations in the neural correlates of reward and motivational processing. These alterations may provoke relapse during early nicotine withdrawal as only nicotine is capable of normalizing DA in these brain regions.

11.3 Cognition

Chapter 4 introduced the concept of cognitive control and its impairment in addiction. Cognitive control processes include a broad class of mental operations, including planning, response inhibition, and action monitoring, and evidence is continually emerging regarding the contributions of the prefrontal cortex (PFC) as a substrate of cognitive control processes. Smoking relapse partly reflects withdrawal, which includes difficulty concentrating and other problems with cognitive control, and these effects can be reversed by cigarette smoking. Effective everyday mental functioning requires cognitive control, and disturbances to cognition during nicotine abstinence may increase the susceptibility to smoking relapse because the control over smoking urges and behaviour is diminished. The ability to monitor one's behaviour within a certain environment during acute nicotine abstinence may be essential when there is a need to detect conflicting circumstances and resolve them quickly, in order to prevent relapse. Indeed, neural functioning during nicotine abstinence in brain regions has actually been shown to be increased under conditions of cognitive control, and may reflect compensatory and adaptive processes in order to cope with the effects of withdrawal. Studies have shown an exaggerated pattern of neural activity in brain regions associated with cognitive control, an effect that remits under conditions of nicotine satiety.

Azizian and colleagues (2010), for example, were able to show that, under conditions of cognitive response conflict, overnight (>12 h) nicotine abstinence induced greater anterior cingulate cortex (ACC) activity (see Figure 11.3). The same figure shows that after smoking there was greater activity in the middle frontal gyrus (MFG). Therefore, exaggerated neural activity during acute nicotine withdrawal may be a reflection of compensatory mechanisms by which networks expend excessive energy to support selective cognitive control processes, which is resolved upon smoking. This suggests that smokers demonstrate

Figure 11.2 Striatal and prefrontal activation associated with a reward anticipation trial type (money or smoking) X condition (abstinent or non-abstinent) interaction. The right caudate head: 6, 4, 2; F = 23.95, 169 voxels; left caudate head: –4, 6, –2; F = 20.18, 121 voxels; and medial prefrontal cortex: 2, 40, 12; F = 20.60, 194 voxels showed the interaction effect. There was greater activation in these regions during abstinence in response to cues that predicted future cigarette rewards, but greater activation during nonabstinence (satiety) in response to cues that predicted future monetary rewards.

Reprinted from *Biological Psychiatry*, 76, 9, Sweitzer, M. M., Geier, C. F., Joel, D.L., et al., Dissociated effects of anticipating smoking versus monetary reward in the caudate as

(a)

(b)

Figure 11.3 Showing that smokers had a significantly greater response during the no-smoking compared smoking session in (a) the anterior cingulate cortex (ACC—*p* <0.02, paired *t*-test), but a significantly greater response during the smoking compared no-smoking session in (b) the middle frontal gyrus (MFG—*p* <0.003, paired *t*-test). The scale represents the colour (from dark to light yellow) of the cluster corresponding to the increasing Z-statistic. The structural image represents the MNI152 average normal brain with corresponding coronal (anterior–posterior) and sagittal (right–left) coordinates.

Reprinted by permission from Macmillan Publishers Ltd: *Neuropsychopharmacology*, 35, 3, Azizian, A., Nestor, L. J., Payer, D. et al., Smoking reduces conflict-related anterior cingulate activity in abstinent cigarette smokers performing a Stroop task, pp. 775–782. Copyright © 2009, Rights managed by Nature Publishing Group.

state-dependent (abstinence vs satiety) alterations in cognition, which are dependent on the functioning of prefrontal brain networks.

Decreased activity in executive brain networks has also been suggested as a marker of relapse. Loughead and colleagues (2015), for example, showed that abstinence-induced decreases in the dorsolateral prefrontal cortex (DLPFC—see Chapter 4) and reduced suppression of the posterior cingulate cortex (PCC) during a working memory task were able to predict smoking relapse, effects that were better than standard clinical variables in predicting treatment outcome (see

Figure 11.4 Whole-brain condition (abstinence challenge, smoking satiety) by group (relapse, quit) ANOVA interaction effect. (B MF/CG and right DLPFC clusters (see above) show comparable activation under the smoking satiety condition in both groups. There is greater activation in the left DLPFC in the smoking satiety condition for the relapse group (vs quit). Under abstinence, challenge signal in all clusters decreases for the relapse group and increases for the quit group. Abbreviations: MF/CG: medial frontal/cingulate gyrus; DLPFC: dorsolateral prefrontal cortex.

Reprinted by permission from Macmillan Publishers Ltd: *Neuropsychopharmacology*, 40, 6, Loughead, J., Wileyto, E. P., Ruparel, K., et al., Working memory-related neural activity predicts future smoking relapse, pp. 1311–1320. Copyright © 2015, Rights Managed by Nature Publishing Group.

Figure 11.4). This suggests that during nicotine abstinence, the ability to activate the DLPFC in situations requiring cognitive control may protect against subsequent relapse. Therefore, the failure to develop, or a loss of previously developed cognitive control in nicotine addiction may affect the ability to restrain cigarette smoking during situations requiring a high degree of cognitive control and self-monitoring. To this end, inferior top-down cognitive control neural processing may be an important factor in provoking smoking relapse as a result of increased, overriding bottom-up neural functioning that biases the choice to reinitiate cigarette smoking.

11.4 Treatments

As supported with empirical evidence, nicotine addiction presents a serious risk to health because of disturbances in brain functioning underlying key behavioural processes—disturbances that promote continued nicotine use. Therefore, treatments that target disruptions to the neural substrates of these processes are likely to improve treatment outcome in nicotine addiction. One such treatment that has been developed for nicotine addiction is varenicline (Chantix). Varenicline is a partial agonist at α4β2 nAChRs (see Chapter 6), and so mimics the effects of nicotine, but to a lesser extent, and also blocks the effects of smoking. Varenicline has been shown to be one of the leading medications for promoting long-term smoking cessation. Evidence suggests that this effect is most likely due to it reducing neural responses to smoking cues, concomitant with attenuated craving.

Franklin and colleagues (2011), for example, were able to show that three weeks of varenicline treatment (compared with placebo) significantly reduced cigarette craving, together with activity in the orbitofrontal cortex (OFC) in response to smoking cues. The OFC was introduced in Chapter 4 in the context of motivation and drive—the goal-directed pursuit of rewards. The OFC is connected with brain regions involved in DA-dependent reinforcement, such as the NAcc, and receives direct DA projections from the midbrain VTA. Importantly, the OFC is involved in the attribution of salience to reinforcing stimuli, and is an established neural correlate that responds to drug cues. Therefore, varenicline's clinical efficacy may surround its attenuating effect on the reward-evaluating processes of the OFC in response to smoking cues. Brandon and colleagues (2011) also reported that varenicline, compared with placebo, reduced tonic and cue-provoked craving, as well as the expected value of cigarettes, the time spent smoking, and self-reported reward (i.e. satisfaction) from cigarette smoking (see Figure 11.5).

Cognitive disturbances are a core symptom of nicotine withdrawal, and as reported, contribute to smoking relapse. Varenicline has also been shown to increase cognitive control-related brain activity during nicotine abstinence (Loughead et al. 2010). These effects were reported in the dorsal anterior cingulate/medial frontal cortex and DLPFC during a working memory task, particularly at high levels of task difficulty, with associated improvements in cognitive performance among those who were heavily nicotine dependent (see Figure 11.6).

Bupropion (see Chapter 7) is a DA reuptake inhibitor and a weak releasing agent that increases the ability to quit smoking, due to its attenuation of withdrawal symptoms. Smokers treated with bupropion describe a reduction in nicotine withdrawal symptoms that include negative affect, the urge to smoke (craving), difficulty concentrating, and irritability. Several studies have now reliably replicated the success of bupropion treatment in smokers, suggesting a common mechanism by which this medication facilitates smoking cessation.

Figure 11.5 Comparison of varenicline (solid line) versus placebo (dotted line) across sessions on (a) tonic craving (Questionnaire of Smoking Urges, total score); (b) cue-provoked craving (ratings in response to smoking images, controlling for neutral images); (c) expected reinforcement value (cigarette choice procedure cross-over value) before the full cigarette; (d) total time smoking (seconds); (e) total number of puffs smoked; and (f) perceived reward (mCEQ: Modified Cigarette Evaluation Questionnaire Satisfaction Scale) following the full cigarette. Error bars indicate standard error. $*p < 0.05$; $**p < 0.01$; $***p < 0.001$.

Reproduced from *Psychopharmacology*, 218, 2, Brandon, T. H., Drobes, D. J., Unrod, M. et al, Varenicline effects on craving, cue reactivity, and smoking reward, pp. 391–403. Copyright © 2011, Springer-Verlag.

One mechanism by which buproprion promotes abstinence is through its ability to attenuate craving and its neural correlates. Culbertson and colleagues (2011) showed that bupropion-treated participants reported less craving, together with less activation in the VS, OFC, and ACC when actively resisting craving, compared with placebo-treated participants. This study also reported

Figure 11.6 Visual N-back working memory task. (a) Coloured regions represent functionally defined ROI masks identified using a whole-brain repeated-measures ANOVA. (b) Mean percent signal change for the 1-back, 2-back, and 3-back conditions from the ROIs. Main effects of treatment (varenicline, placebo) were observed in all three ROIs, significant at $p < 0.05$; DLPFC, dorsolateral prefrontal cortex; MF/CG, dorsal anterior cingulate/medial frontal cortex; ROI, region of interest; BOLD, blood oxygenation level-dependent.

Reprinted from Biological Psychiatry, 67, 8, Loughhead, J., Ray, R.., Wileyto, E. P. et al., Effects of the alpha4beta2 partial agonist varenicline on brain activity and working memory in abstinent smokers, pp. 715–721. Copyright © 2010 Society of Biological Psychiatry. Published by Elsevier Inc. All rights reserved.

that reductions in self-reported craving correlated with reduced activation in these brain regions. Interestingly, bupropion also acts as a weak antagonist at nAChRs, decreasing the probability of their activation by nicotine. Therefore, bupropion may also reduce the reinforcing value of smoking should patients relapse during treatment.

The effects of bupropion on smoking cessation may also include improvements in cognitive processing during nicotine abstinence which as discussed, is a potential prognostic marker of relapse. Perkins and colleagues (2013) has shown that, compared with placebo, bupropion during early smoking abstinence significantly improves working memory performance (see Figure 11.7). The DLPFC is particularly involved in the 'on-line' processing of information (i.e. working memory), and is in receipt of DA projections from the midbrain VTA. Importantly, DA activity in the DLPFC is involved in the modulation of cognitive control processes, perhaps suggesting that the efficacy of bupropion to improve cognitive processing in nicotine abstinence is due to its dopaminergic effects in this region.

One other potential benefit of bupropion for smokers is that it also has antidepressant effects—indeed, this was its first medical use. When people smoke tobacco become addicted to the nicotine, there are also chemicals in the burning tobacco that block the enzyme called monoamine oxidase (MOA). This enzyme breaks down DA, serotonin, and noradrenaline, which means smoking can elevate levels of these neurotransmitters. Fowler and colleagues (1996) indeed reported that the brains of living smokers show a 40% decrease in the level of MAO-B compared to non-smokers or former smokers. MAO-B is specifically involved in the breakdown of DA, which as discussed throughout this volume, is a neurotransmitter implicated in reward and motivation. Upon smoking cessation, however, MAO blockade by tobacco is lifted, so the enzyme then resumes its breaking-down activity of these neurotransmitters. Therefore, increased MAO activity in potentially deficient neurotransmitter systems in nicotine addiction, contributes to the low mood many smokers experience when they initially quit. Bupropion, by enhancing DA and noradrenaline, offsets this deficit to some extent. Recently we have seen in many countries the rise of e-cigarettes (e-cigs) or vaping. Here a nicotine solution is heated and inhaled. This provides the brain with nicotine to counteract the deficit seen in tobacco withdrawal. As vaping liquids are much less toxic than burning tobacco (see Nutt et al. 2014), vaping is seen as a powerful means of tobacco harm reduction.

11.5 Conclusion

The majority of cigarette smokers endorse the desire to give up smoking but only a small percentage will ever achieve full nicotine abstinence. Despite their best efforts and expressed preferences, nicotine-dependent individuals often appear

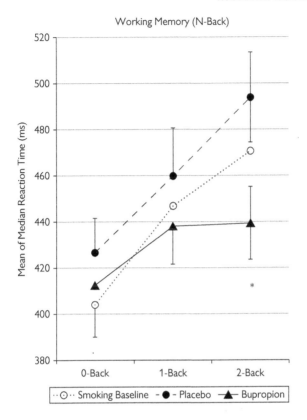

Figure 11.7 Mean±SE of the median response time for correct responses on N-back task of working memory, by memory load, during initial smoking baseline to learn the task and due to placebo or bupropion after overnight tobacco abstinence (N = 24). * p = 0.01 for the difference between bupropion and placebo in responding to 2-back vs 0-back.

Reprinted from *Drug and Alcohol Dependence*, 133, 1, Perkins, K. A., Karelitz, J. L., Jao, N. C., et al., Effects of bupropion on cognitive performance during initial tobacco abstinence, pp. 283–286. Copyright © 2013 Elsevier Ireland Ltd. All rights reserved.

incapable of exerting sufficient control over their smoking urges and behaviour. This inability to exert control appears to implicate potential disturbances in reward processing, salience attribution, and ultimately, diminished cognitive control. Importantly, treatments that attenuate disturbances to reward and cognitive networks in the brain, particular during early abstinence, are conferred with the efficacy to promote smoking cessation and protect against relapse.

REFERENCES AND FURTHER READING

Azizian A, Nestor LJ, Payer D, et al. (2010). Smoking reduces conflict-related anterior cingulate activity in abstinent cigarette smokers performing a stroop task. *Neuropsychopharmacology*, **35**(3), 775–82. doi:10.1038/npp.2009.186.

Brandon TH, Drobes DJ, Unrod M, et al. (2011). Varenicline effects on craving, cue reactivity, and smoking reward. *Psychopharmacology (Berl)*, **218**(2), 391–403.

Brody AL, Olmstead RE, London ED, et al. (2004). Smoking-induced ventral striatum dopamine release. *American Journal of Psychiatry*, **161**(7), 1211–18.

Brody AL, Mandelkern MA, London ED, et al. (2006a). Cigarette smoking saturates brain alpha 4 beta 2 nicotinic acetylcholine receptors. *Archives of General Psychiatry*, **63**(8), 907–15.

Brody AL, Mandelkern MA, Olmstead RE, et al. (2006b). Gene variants of brain dopamine pathways and smoking-induced dopamine release in the ventral caudate/nucleus accumbens. *Archives of General Psychiatry*, **63**(7), 808–16. doi:10.1001/archpsyc.63.7.808.

Brody AL, Mukhin AG, Stephanie S, et al. (2013). Treatment for tobacco dependence: effect on brain nicotinic acetylcholine receptor density. *Neuropsychopharmacology*, **38**(8), 1548–56. doi:10.1038/npp.2013.53.

Culbertson CS, Bramen J, Cohen MS, et al. (2011). Effect of bupropion treatment on brain activation induced by cigarette-related cues in smokers. *Archives of General Psychiatry*, **68**(5), 505–15.

Feduccia AA, Chatterjee S, and Bartlett SE (2012). Neuronal nicotinic acetylcholine receptors: neuroplastic changes underlying alcohol and nicotine addictions. *Frontiers in Molecular Neuroscience*, **5**, 83. doi:10.3389/fnmol.2012.00083.

Fehr C, Yakushev I, Hohmann N, et al. (2008). Association of low striatal dopamine d2 receptor availability with nicotine dependence similar to that seen with other drugs of abuse. *American Journal of Psychiatry*, **165**(4), 507–14.

Fowler JS, Volkow ND, Wang GJ, et al. (1996). Inhibition of monoamine oxidase B in the brains of smokers. *Nature*, **379**(6567), 733–6. doi:10.1038/379733a0.

Franklin T, Wang Z, Suh JJ, et al. (2011). Effects of varenicline on smoking cue-triggered neural and craving responses. *Archives of General Psychiatry*, **68**(5), 516–26.

Loughead J, Wileyto EP, Ruparel K, et al. (2015). Working memory-related neural activity predicts future smoking relapse. *Neuropsychopharmacology*, **40**(6), 1311–20.

Loughead J, Ray R, Wileyto EP, et al. (2010). Effects of the alpha4beta2 partial agonist varenicline on brain activity and working memory in abstinent smokers. *Biological Psychiatry*, **67**(8), 715–21.

Nutt DJ, Phillips LD, Balfour D, et al. (2014). Estimating the Harms of Nicotine-Containing Products Using the MCDA Approach. *European Addiction Research*, **20**(5), 218–25. doi:10.1159/000360220.

Perkins KA, Karelitz JL, Jao NC, et al. (2013). Effects of bupropion on cognitive performance during initial tobacco abstinence. *Drug and Alcohol Dependency*, **133**(1), 283–6.

Rose EJ, Ross TJ, Salmeron BJ, et al. (2011). Chronic exposure to nicotine is associated with reduced reward-related activity in the striatum but not the midbrain. *Biological Psychiatry*, **71**(3), 206–13.

Sweitzer MM, Geier CF, Joel DL, et al. (2014). Dissociated effects of anticipating smoking versus monetary reward in the caudate as a function of smoking abstinence. *Biological Psychiatry*, **76**(9), 681–8. doi:10.1016/j.biopsych.2013.11.013.

Appetite hormones and addiction

KEY POINTS

- Appetite and feeding are regulated by hormones that affect the brain.
- These hormones signal the present energy state of the body.
- These hormones can regulate reward and motivational processes.
- Ghrelin is an orexigenic gut hormone that activates reward circuitry.
- Ghrelin increase the consumption of food, but also drugs of addiction.
- Glucagon-like peptide-1 (GLP-1) is an anorexigenic hormone.
- GLP-1 reduces the consumption of food and drugs of addiction.
- Treatments that regulate appetite hormones and their receptors are viable targets for preventing relapse in addiction disorders.

Throughout this volume we have discussed evidence that addiction is characterized by the compulsion to seek and take a substance, the loss of control in limiting substance intake, and the emergence of a negative emotional state (e.g. dysphoria, anxiety) when intake is prevented (see Chapter 4). Importantly, this addiction trajectory is a reflection of functional disturbances to brain networks involved in controlling necessary motivational and cognitive processes (see Chapter 4—key neural substrates). Intriguingly, many of these same behavioural and brain disturbances are also seen in patients with obesity and binge-eating disorder (BED), suggesting that there are shared neural substrates between substance addiction and compulsive food consumption. Therefore, addiction and atypical eating behaviours (as seen in obesity and BED) may share some of their aetiology due to the effects of certain appetite hormones on the neural circuitry that supports reward, motivation, and cognition.

Food intake and appetite are regulated by numerous circulating hormones and neuropeptides, which signal the present energy state of the body. These signals are received by the brain, particularly the hypothalamus, eliciting the appropriate physiological responses to feed and restore energy. Several of these hormones, however, have also been shown to target brain areas implicated in reward processing, and significantly, addiction. Therefore, the possibility that endocrine signals from the gut traditionally known to regulate food intake, energy, and body weight homeostasis may also play a role in the regulation of reward and motivational processes should now be considered, in light of emerging evidence for their modulating effects on other types of behaviours.

12.1 Appetite hormones

Ghrelin is a 28 amino acid stomach-derived peptide hormone that activates hypothalamic orexigenic neurons, and inhibits anorectic (appetite-suppressing) neurons, to induce hunger and stimulate feeding. Ghrelin is an endogenous ligand at the growth hormone secretagogue receptor (GHS-R1a). GHS-R1a receptors are highly co-expressed with dopamine (DA) receptors in the midbrain, suggesting a modulatory role in reward processing. Specifically, it is thought that ghrelin activates cholinergic projections from the lateral dorsal tegmental nucleus (LDTg) in the brainstem, and these neurons project to release acetylcholine (ACh) onto nicotinic receptors ($\alpha 3 \beta 2$, $\beta 3$, and $\alpha 6$) on DA neurons of the VTA. Ghrelin administration in humans has been shown to provoke neural responses associated with reward. Malik and colleagues (2008), for example, showed that ghrelin administered intravenously to healthy volunteers during fMRI increased neural responses to food pictures in a number of brain regions, including the amygdala, orbitofrontal cortex (OFC), anterior insula cortex, and striatum—brain regions that are implicated in encoding the incentive value of food cues (see Figure 12.1). These effects of ghrelin in the amygdala and OFC were also found to be correlated with self-rated hunger scores, suggesting that ghrelin enhances hedonic responses to food-related cues. Similar effects have also been reported by Goldstone and colleagues (2014) in the hippocampus and OFC. Therefore, there is strong evidence that ghrelin activates corticolimbic DA circuitry in the presence of food cues, suggesting that it may also play a modulating role in other types of rewards.

In preclinical studies, ghrelin (and food restriction) have indeed been shown to increase consumptive and reward behaviours to nicotine, alcohol, cocaine, and other drugs of abuse, as well as food. Preliminary studies in humans show differences in endogenous blood ghrelin levels in actively drinking and abstinent alcoholics. For example, Leggio and colleagues (2012) found significant differences in blood ghrelin between non-abstinent and abstinent alcoholics that were significantly and positively correlated with alcohol craving (see Figure 12.2). Other studies also indicate a significant positive correlation between ghrelin levels and alcohol craving, suggesting that this hormone may mediate the urge to drink alcohol due to its effects on mesolimbic DA circuitry. Leggio and colleagues (2012) administered intravenous ghrelin (1mcg/kg, 3 mcg/kg, or 0 mcg/kg placebo) to alcoholics, followed by a cue reactivity procedure—participants were exposed to neutral (juice) and alcohol cues. This study showed that during ghrelin (3 mcg/kg vs placebo) craving was significantly increased for alcohol (but not juice), providing strong preliminary evidence that ghrelin directly mediates alcohol craving (see Figure 12.3). Taken together, the effects of the ghrelin system in response to food and drug cues suggest that this orexigenic gut hormone is a powerful mediator of reward. Despite the scarcity of research, the few studies that have been conducted appear to demonstrate that the ghrelin system may be a viable target

Figure 12.1 (a) Activation maps for amygdala, fusiform gyrus, insula, pulvinar, and OFC regions when viewing food images during ghrelin administration. Arrows indicate the peak locations within each brain region. (b) Bar graph showing the BOLD activation in the ghrelin and control conditions for different regions identified. All comparisons show a significant effect of ghrelin (p < 0.0001, two-tailed). Error bars represent the SD. (c) Correlation between mean self-ratings of hunger during the ghrelin scans and the change in BOLD activation due to ghrelin. Abbreviations: OFC: orbitofrontal cortex; SN/VTA: substantia nigra, ventral tegmental area; Ins: insula.

Reprinted from Cell Metabolism, 75, S, Malik, S., McGlone, F., Bedrossian, D. et al., Ghrelin modulates brain activity in areas that control appetitive behavior. pp. 400–409.

CHAPTER 12

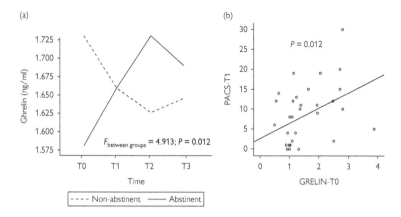

Figure 12.2 (a) Ghrelin changes of subjects who were abstinent versus those who were not abstinent during a 12-week period. There was a statistical difference in the changes of ghrelin between the two groups ($F = 4.913$, $P = 0.012$). (b) Relationship between baseline ghrelin levels (Ghrelin-T0) and Penn Alcohol Craving Scale (PACS) scores at T1. Ghrelin-T0 was significantly and positively correlated with the PACS score at T1 ($r = 0.423$, $P = 0.012$). PACS = Penn Alcohol Craving Scale.

Reproduced from *Addiction Biology*, 7, 2, Leggio, L., Ferrulli, A., Cardone, S. et al., Ghrelin system in alcohol-dependent subjects: role of plasma ghrelin levels in alcohol drinking and craving, pp. 452–464. © 2011 The Authors, Addiction Biology © 2011 Society for the Study of Addiction, published by John Wiley and Sons 2012.

for ameliorating behaviours related to compulsive consumption, including drug and alcohol addiction.

The **orexin** (or hypocretin) system is made up of two neuropeptides, which include orexin-A and orexin-B. Orexin is produced from prepro-orexin in the lateral hypothalamus. **Orexin-A** is a 33 amino-acid neuropeptide and is an agonist at both Ox_1 and Ox_2 receptors. **Orexin-B** is a 28 amino-acid neuropeptide, which only activates Ox_2 receptors. Orexin neurons project widely throughout the central nervous system, with their receptors expressed in the cerebral cortex, the striatum, and VTA. The orexin system is involved in a variety of processes such as arousal, reward, energy homeostasis, and cognition. Evidence is now emerging, however, that the orexin system may also have a role to play in addiction.

The orexigenic neuropeptides (both types A and B) have recently been shown to promote alcohol intake, and also affect craving, withdrawal, and relapse to drugs of addiction. Intra-VTA application of the orexin-A peptide increases cocaine-seeking behaviour and enhances cocaine-evoked increases in DA transmission to ventral striatal targets. Blockade of orexin transmission appears to reduce the reinforcing effects of cocaine by attenuating DA

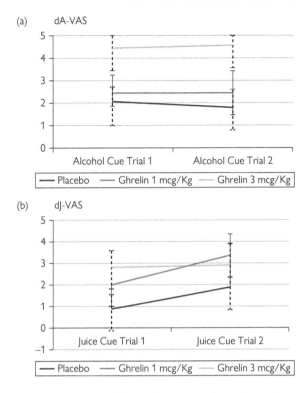

Figure 12.3 (a) Increase in alcohol urge by dose, expressed as its increase compared to the baseline (pre-drug) value of the Alcohol-Visual Analogue Scale (dA-VAS). Analyses indicated that ghrelin dose was statistically related to alcohol urge increase [$F(2,40) = 3.36$, $p = 0.045$], and Bonferroni-corrected pairwise comparisons revealed that alcohol urge was significantly greater for ghrelin 3 mcg/kg than placebo ($p = 0.046$). The effect size for the increase in alcohol urge for ghrelin 3 mcg/kg versus placebo was large ($d = 0.94$). (b) Increase in juice urge by dose, expressed as its increase compared to the baseline (pre-drug) value of the Juice-Visual Analogue Scale (dJ-VAS). Analyses indicated that ghrelin dose was not statistically related to juice urge increase [$F(2,40) = 1.16$, $p = 0.32$].

Reprinted from *Biological Psychiatry*, 76, 9, Leggio, L., Zywiak, W.H., Fricchione, S.R., et al., Intravenous ghrelin administration increases alcohol craving in alcohol-dependent heavy drinkers: a preliminary investigation, pp. 734–741. Copyright © 2014 Elsevier.

transmission in the VTA, with OX_1 receptor antagonists attenuating cued and stress-induced reinstatement of cocaine-seeking. Thus, orexin transmission appears to mediate aspects of the rewarding and reinforcing properties of addictive drugs through both receptor subtypes, with antagonists reducing these effects. Research in humans by Ziółkowski and colleagues (2016) have also shown that orexin blood concentrations are significantly higher in alcohol-dependent patients, and that after four weeks of treatment for relapse prevention, these levels decrease significantly to a similar value observed in a comparison control group (see Figure 12.4). This study also showed that those with a higher level of alcohol dependence had the highest orexin blood concentrations at the beginning of treatment which after four weeks diminished to the same level as those seen in patients with less severe dependence. Therefore, given the role orexin appears to play in the motivation for drug rewards, it (or its receptor) may represent a potential target for relapse prevention treatment in alcohol and cocaine addiction.

Glucagon-like peptide-l (GLP-1) is an anorexigenic peptide hormone released from intestinal L-cells after feeding. GLP-1 increases insulin secretion in a glucose-dependent manner, improves insulin sensitivity, and increases satiety by delaying gastric emptying. The effects of GLP-1 in the brain are believed to be through its hypothalamic–brainstem actions that reduce appetite and food intake. In preclinical studies GLP-1 agonists decrease both consumption and the rewarding value of food through its actions on mesolimbic DA pathways. Anorexigenic hormones, including GLP-1, also attenuate reward system responses to food in human fMRI studies. Gastric bypass surgery, known to increase GLP-1, has been shown to reduce brain responses to high calorie foods in obese subjects, particularly in the OFC, amygdala, striatum, and hippocampus (see Figure 12.5). This appears to lend credence to the supposition that augmenting GLP-1 reduces the incentive value of food reward.

Research by van Bloemendaal and colleagues (2014) showed that the GLP-1 receptor agonist exenatide (currently used for the treatment of type 2 diabetes to stimulate satiety) reduced activation in appetite- and reward-related brain regions when viewing food pictures. The effects of GLP-1 receptor activation, it has been suggested, are to decrease the prediction of food reward, but increase the hedonic response to food, which may reduce craving and prevent overeating respectively. Indeed, van Bloemendaal and colleagues (2015) have also shown that exenatide, compared to placebo, decreases neural responses to the anticipation of a high calorie reward (chocolate milk), but increases neural responses to the receipt of the reward (see Figures 12.6 and 12.7 respectively). These neural responses were also paralleled by reductions in food intake. Therefore, GLP-1 agonists, such as exenatide, may reduce the hedonic threshold during food consumption, which means there is a greater and more rapid satiation during eating. This effect then prevents overeating to compensate for the original blunted hedonic response. This may also suggest that the GLP-1 system is another viable target for remediating behaviours related to the compulsive consumption of drugs. Indeed, recent preclinical studies using GLP-1 agonists in animal models have been reported to reduce alcohol, nicotine, cocaine and stimulant reward (e.g. conditioned place preference), drug-induced accumbal DA release, and drug consumption.

Figure 12.4 (a) Blood orexin concentration at the start of the study and after a four-week period of abstinence in alcohol-dependent patients and in the control group. ANOVA: $F(1, 53) = 4.90$; $P = 0.031$; *$P < 0.01$ in relation to the initial value obtained in alcohol-dependent patients. (b) Blood orexin concentration at the start of the study and after a four-week period of abstinence in relation to the Short Alcohol Dependence Data (SADD) score range for moderate and heavy alcohol dependence. ANOVA: $F(1, 26) = 6.75$; $P = 0.015$; *$P < 0.05$-statistical significance of difference between the initial values in both groups and between the initial and after 4-week treatment in patients with the initial SADD score 20–45.

Reproduced from *Alcohol and Alcoholism*, 51, 4, Ziolkowski, M., Czarnecki, D., Budzynski, J., et al., Orexin in Patients with Alcohol Dependence Treated for Relapse Prevention: A Pilot Study, pp. 416–421. © The Author 2015. Medical Council on Alcohol and Oxford University Press. All rights reserved.

Figure 12.5 Whole brain comparison of activation to high-calorie foods where obese patients after gastric bypass (RYGB) and showed significantly less activation than patients after gastric banding (BAND). No clusters showed greater activation in RYGB than BAND groups. Colour bar indicates Z values. Abbreviations: ACC: anterior cingulate cortex, Amy: amygdala, Caud: caudate, NAcc: nucleus accumbens, Hipp: hippocampus, MFG: middle frontal gyrus, OFC: orbitofrontal cortex, Put: putamen.

12.2 Treatments

The role of appetite hormones in reward and motivation has potential therapeutic implications for the future management of addiction. Given that GLP-1 analogues, such as exenatide, are now approved for type 2 diabetes, GLP-1 analogues could conceivably be used in the treatment of drug dependence. Presently, however, these treatments are not licensed for addiction disorders, but there are ongoing trials in human addiction populations which are aiming to elucidate the potential efficacy of exenatide in addiction disorders. Likewise, there are ongoing studies in human addiction investigating the potential efficacy of ghrelin receptor antagonism, given some of the preclinical evidence that this may also be a viable target for treating disorders of compulsive consumption, particularly alcoholism. There are also ongoing studies investigating the efficacy of orexin antagonists for addiction disorders. Suvorexant, for example, which is a dual orexin receptor antagonist (and FDA-approved to treat insomnia), has recently been shown to

Figure 12.6 Effects of glucagon-like peptide-1 (GLP-1) receptor activation on brain responses to anticipatory food reward. Coronal slices showing brain regions where exenatide vs placebo reduced brain activation in (a) lean subjects and (b) subjects with type 2 diabetes in response to anticipatory food reward (anticipation to receipt of chocolate milk vs tasteless solution). Left side of the coronal slices is the left side of the brain. Y is the Montreal Neurological Institute space Y coordinate of the axial slice. The colour scale reflects the T value of the functional activity. In the graphs BOLD signal intensity (effect size) for the different test days is plotted (arbitrary units), mean and standard error of the mean. EXE, exenatide; OFC, orbitofrontal cortex.

Reproduced from Diabetes, Obesity and Metabolism, 17, 9, Van Bloemendaal, L., Veltman, D.J., Ten Kulve, J.S., et al., Brain reward-system activation in response to anticipation and consumption of palatable food is altered by glucagon-like peptide-1 receptor activation in humans, pp. 878–886. © 2015 John Wiley & Sons Ltd.

Figure 12.7 Effects of glucagon-like peptide-1 (GLP-1) receptor activation on brain responses to consummatory food reward. Coronal slices showing brain regions where exenatide versus placebo increased brain activation in (a) lean subjects, (b) obese subjects and (c) subjects with type 2 diabetes in response to consummatory food reward (chocolate milk vs tasteless solution). Left side of the coronal slices is the left side of the brain. Y is the Montreal Neurological Institute space Y coordinate of the axial slice. The colour scale reflects the T value of the functional activity. In the graphs BOLD signal intensity (effect size) for the different test days is plotted (arbitrary units), mean and standard error of the mean. EXE, exenatide; OFC, orbitofrontal cortex.

Reproduced from *Diabetes, Obesity and Metabolism*, 17, 9, Van Bloemendaal, L., Veltman, D.J., Ten Kulve, J.S., et al., Brain reward-system activation in response to anticipation and consumption of palatable food is altered by glucagon-like peptide-1 receptor activation in humans, pp. 878–886. © 2015 John Wiley & Sons Ltd.

reduce cocaine administration and attenuate cocaine-induced elevations in ventral striatal DA in animals (see Gentile et al. 2017). While only preliminary, these types of research findings using a medication approved for use in humans bestow some optimism for the value of exploring brain endocrine pathways in the treatment of addiction disorders.

12.3 Conclusion

There is now evidence in animals that some appetite hormones influence the consumption of and desire for food, and also the intake of drugs of addiction. The two best examples, given some of the preclinical findings, are GLP1 and ghrelin, but there are other candidate systems (orexins) that are emerging as viable targets. The influence of these hormones is exerted through brain systems involved in the core behavioural components of addiction: reward sensitivity, stress, impulsivity and compulsivity. These behavioural components are also seen in obesity and BED. It is unknown whether these hormones directly influence the core behavioural components of addiction in humans, particularly during abstinence, but new research is attempting to address this. Therefore, there is an emerging shift into a new field of testing drugs that affect appetite hormones and their receptors, and their use in regulating the brain mechanisms that lead to relapse in addiction disorders.

REFERENCES AND FURTHER READING

Engel JA and Jerlhag E (2014). Role of appetite-regulating peptides in the pathophysiology of addiction: implications for pharmacotherapy. *CNS Drugs*, **28**(10), 875–6.

Gentile TA, Simmons SJ, Barker DJ, et al. (2017). Suvorexant, an orexin/hypocretin receptor antagonist, attenuates motivational and hedonic properties of cocaine. *Addiction Biology*. doi:10.1111/adb.12507.

Goldstone AP, Prechtl CG, Scholtz S, et al. (2014). Ghrelin mimics fasting to enhance human hedonic, orbitofrontal cortex, and hippocampal responses to food. *American Journal of Clinical Nutrition*, **99**(6), 1319–30.

Leggio L, Ferrulli A, Cardone S, et al. (2012). Ghrelin system in alcohol-dependent subjects: role of plasma ghrelin levels in alcohol drinking and craving. *Addiction Biology*, **17**(2), 452–64. doi:10.1111/j.1369–1600.2010.00308.x.

Malik S, McGlone F, Bedrossian D, et al. (2008). Ghrelin modulates brain activity in areas that control appetitive behavior. *Cell Metabolism*, **7**(5), 400–9.

Scholtz S, Miras AD, Chhina N, et al. (2014). Obese patients after gastric bypass surgery have lower brain-hedonic responses to food than after gastric banding. *Gut*, **63**(6), 891–902.

van Bloemendaal L, Ijzerman RG, Ten Kulve JS, et al. (2014). GLP-1 receptor activation modulates appetite- and reward-related brain areas in humans. *Diabetes*, **63**(12), 4186–96.

van Bloemendaal L, Veltman DJ, Ten Kulve JS, et al. (2015). Brain reward-system activation in response to anticipation and consumption of palatable food is altered by glucagon-like peptide-1 receptor activation in humans, *Diabetes, Obesity and Metabolism*, **17**(9), 878–86.

Ziółkowski M, Czarnecki D, Budzynski J, et al. (2016). Orexin in patients with alcohol dependence treated for relapse prevention: a pilot study. *Alcohol and Alcoholism*, **51**(4), 416–21. doi:10.1093/alcalc/agv129.

CHAPTER 13

Conclusion and overview

KEY POINTS

- Substances of addiction are highly reinforcing because they induce pleasure.
- Cocaine and amphetamines trigger exaggerated increases in dopamine.
- GABA is the major inhibitory neurotransmitter in the brain.
- Compounds that target the GABA system may help in the treatment of addiction.
- Addiction involves glutamate-dependent neuroplasticity in the brain.
- Medications that target glutamate may be efficacious in preventing drug relapse.
- The brain contains a complex system of endogenous opioid peptides.
- The mu opioid receptor appears to be involved in substance abuse and addiction.
- Compounds that target the mu opioid receptor system may help treat addiction.
- Nicotine causes disturbances in reward and cognitive processing.
- Smoking cessation medications are available to treat nicotine addiction.
- Appetite and feeding are regulated by hormones that affect the brain.
- These hormones can regulate reward and motivational processes.
- Treatments that regulate appetite hormones could treat addiction disorders.
- Some individuals may be more susceptible to substance addiction than others.

Substance addiction is a chronic relapsing disorder. Individuals abuse substances for different reasons. There may be personal and mitigating circumstances that lead people to substance abuse (e.g. stress or unhappiness). People may also be at increased risk of initiating substance abuse due to their age. The commencement of adolescence, for example, is a unique period of neurobiological development. Compared to children and adults, adolescents exhibit a number of psychological traits, such as risky and reward-seeking behaviour. The emergence of these traits may reflect the relatively early functional development of brain limbic affective and reward systems compared to the prefrontal cortex. As such, the period of adolescence may confer a vulnerability to the onset of drug misuse and addiction due to developmental changes in neurobiology, which seem to encourage reward-centred and risky decision-making behaviour.

Additionally, there are genetic risks for substance abuse. Twin registry and adoption studies, for example, have shown that the heritability of alcoholism may be as high as 50–60%. Whatever the cause, substance abuse and dependence confers significant social, mental, and medical impairment in those individuals af-flicted, together with huge economic costs to society.

Substance abuse and dependence is the manifestation of the long-term pharmacological actions of substances on the receptor mechanisms of the brain's neural circuitry. Recent research, however, is beginning to reveal that non-drug or behavioural addictions, especially gambling, show strong neural similarities to substance addiction. Therefore, research examining the brains of both substance and behavioural addiction populations are likely to elucidate what the effects of substances of abuse are on the brain as well as the common processes underpin-ning addiction as whole.

We have discussed the possible role of different neurotransmitter systems in substance abuse and addiction—particularly their role in modulating various elements in the addiction cycle (see Figure 13.1). We have additionally learned that in nicotine addiction, obesity, and BED there exist the same disturbances in reward processing, salience attribution, and cognitive control—similar to other types of addictions. We have additionally learned that endocrine signals, trad-itionally known to regulate food intake and energy homeostasis, may also play a role in the regulation of reward and motivational processes. Importantly, there is an emerging shift into a new field of testing drugs that affect appetite hormones and their receptors, and their use in regulating the brain mechanisms that modu-late relapse in addiction disorders.

The precise roles of these neurotransmitter and hormonal systems and their collective roles in addiction, however, remain equivocal. These findings can ex-plain the mode of action of many current treatments of addiction and also offer the possibility of new therapies. Moreover, although addiction is a recurrent

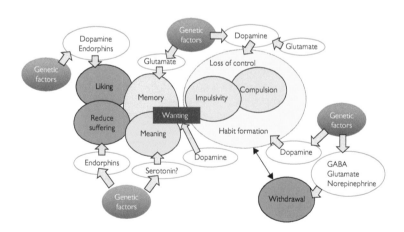

Figure 13.1 **Key elements of addiction and their neurochemical basis. The neuro-chemistry of these elements is likely influenced by individual genetic factors.**

disorder that is difficult to cure, treatments do possess efficacy to aiding people to remaining abstinent, which helps patients stabilize their lives to accommodate other potential courses of treatment (e.g. cognitive–behavioural).

The uncertainty surrounding the role of different neurotransmitter systems in substance abuse and dependence is further complicated by research revealing numerous genetic polymorphisms in these systems—polymorphisms in the dopamine and opioid systems of the brain have been shown to moderate the efficacy of medications to treat and manage substance addiction. Substance addiction, therefore, is a complex disease whose onset, persistence, and treatment are likely influenced by interactions between genetic, environmental, and pharmacological factors.

CHAPTER 13

Index

Tables, figures, and boxes are indicated by an italic *t*, *f*, and *b* following the page number.